TECHNOLOGY AND THE WELFARE STATE

The influence of technological change
upon the development of health care
in Britain and America

Stephen Uttley

London
UNWIN HYMAN
Boston   Sydney   Wellington

Published by the Academic Division of
Unwin Hyman Ltd
15/17 Broadwick Street, London W1V 1FP, UK

Unwin Hyman Inc.,
955 Massachusetts Avenue, Cambridge, Mass. 02139, USA

Allen & Unwin (Australia) Ltd,
8 Napier Street, North Sydney, NSW 2060, Australia

Allen & Unwin (New Zealand) Ltd
in association with the Port Nicholson Press Ltd
Compusales Building, 75 Ghuznee Street, Wellington 1, New Zealand

First published in 1991

British Library Cataloguing in Publication Data

Uttley, Stephen
    Technology and the welfare state: the development of
    health care in Britain and America.
    1. Welfare work. Applications of computer systems
    I. Title
    361.30385
    ISBN 0–04–445841–X

Library of Congress Cataloging-in-Publication Data

Uttley, Stephen
    Technology and the welfare state: the development of
    health care in Britain and America / Stephen Uttley
        p.   cm.
    Includes bibliographical references and index.
    ISBN 0–04–445840–1 (HB) : $49.95. –
    ISBN 0–04–445841–X (PB) : $17.95.
        1. Social medicine–Great Britain–History–20th century.
        2. Medical care–Great Britain–History–20th century.
        3. Medical technology–Great Britain–History–20th century.
        4. Social Medical–United States– History–20th century.
        5. Medical care–United States–History 20th century.
        6. Medical technology–United States–History–20th century.
        I. Title.
    RA418.3.G7U88   1991   90–41144
    362.1'0425–dc20   CIP

Typeset in 10 on 12 point Bembo
Printed and bound in Great Britain by
Biddles Ltd, Guildford and King's Lynn

Contents

Contents

List of tables

Acknowledgements

I am grateful to my colleagues, both past and present, in the Department of Sociology and Social Work, Victoria University, for their support and in particular I would like to thank Patricia Harris, Bob Tristram and David Pearson. I would especially like to acknowledge the encouragement and assistance which my fellow social policy specialist Avery Jack has given to me over many years of working together and for the example she has set in her own research, writing and teaching. The Council of Victoria University granted me a one year period of research leave during which the initial draft was completed. My thanks to Robert Goodin for his constructive comments at the review stage; these were helpful in planning revisions to the initial manuscript. Gordon Smith of Unwin Hyman has been a source of continual encouragement and help. Last, but by no means least, thanks to my family who have helped me to survive the gestation process for a first-time author. As is always the case the author bears the responsibility for the final product of that process.

Introduction

The welfare state has become a well-established institutional feature of Western industrialized societies. Most member countries of the OECD experienced considerably reduced levels of economic growth in the 1970s and early 1980s. Diminished rates of growth have followed a period of sustained expansion in public social programmes and expenditures. In these circumstances criticisms of the performance, objectives and indeed the future desirability of the welfare state have become part of political and wider public debate. This questioning has led many commentators to label this process of public debate as representing a 'crisis' point in the continuation of the welfare state as we have known it.

Criticisms of the operation of welfare states have focused on how resources are generated and allocated through government-funded or -provided programmes. In relation to how resources are generated, questions are raised about the capacity of the tax base to fund welfare and the likely range of taxpayer responses to an increasing tax burden. Looking at how resources are allocated through welfare state provisions, concern is focused upon what impact social service programmes have had upon levels of well-being in the community in the sense of improved health status, education and the abolition of poverty. Particular attention is paid to the perceived lack of impact of services on those who appear to be most in need of help.

The welfare state involves the transformation of resources into goods and services; that is, it is a production process. Within the debate about crisis in the welfare state consideration of production has largely been confined to questions of political economy. Discussion focuses upon the relative merits of public and private sector provision in terms of efficient resource use and value-questions about consumer freedom and choice. These are important questions but irrespective of our answers to these questions the fact remains that areas such as education, health and income maintenance involve the production of goods and services. One of the ways in which we have sought to under- stand such production in other parts of the economy is through an examination of the technological base of production and how this technology changes over time. This kind of exploration of technological change is conspicuously absent from the theories of welfare state development that are presently available in the social policy literature. This book is based upon the simple proposition that the welfare state does involve the production of goods and services and that examining the technology used in such production and how it has changed over time will contribute to our understanding of particular social services and of the development of the welfare state as a whole.

The book is divided into two parts. Part I consists of a case study of the impact of technological change upon the development of health care systems in Britain and America since the mid-nineteenth century.

Chapter 1 outlines the importance of health care within the welfare state and within the national economies of Britain and America. The chapter includes a review of the general literature on the impact of technology and technological change upon the production of goods and services. Especial attention is paid to the importance of the social context in which innovation occurs and social innovation in the form of organizational and managerial changes.

Chapter 2 involves the construction of a conceptual frame- work for analysing technological change in health care. These various components of health care technology are then examined using the notion that technological change is a dynamic process which includes invention, innovation and diffusion. The chapter concludes with a more detailed examination of how technologi- cal change has impacted upon the rise of the modern hospital, developments in general practice and non-product innovations in the pharmaceutical industry.

Chapter 3 examines the way in which technological change has contributed to changes in the location of health care pro- duction and the exercise of control over services. Technology has an important effect upon how the resources of capital and labour are utilized in a production process. The influence of technological change on the factors of production is described and analysed. Technology affects not only how goods and services are produced but also how they are consumed and these changes are identified. The chapter concludes by looking at possible innovations which may transform the ways in which future health care needs are met.

Chapter 4 focuses upon political innovations which modify the actions of government in terms of direct action as a provider or funder of health care services and indirect actions which affect the conditions under which the health care market operates. The final section examines the argument that the systems of health care provision in America and Britain have tended to become more alike over time.

Chapter 5 assesses claimed links between technological innovation and long term changes in economic activity. The pattern of innovation in health care is tested against available theories and a number of propositions advanced about possible links between different types of innovation and phases in long-wave economic cycles.

Part II of the book consists of a single chapter in which the objective is to apply the findings of the case study of the impact of technological change on the development of health care to an understanding of the welfare state in general. The limitations in the handling of technology in existing accounts for the development of welfare states are described and the main findings of the analysis of health care summarized. The contribution which an understanding of technological change can make to learning about individual social services and the welfare state as a whole is then outlined. The book concludes with an explanation of how such an understanding of technological change casts light on contemporary discussion of 'crisis' in the welfare state.

To Elizabeth, Sarah and Katherine

PART I

Health Care and Technological Change

1 Technological Change and Social Service Production

HEALTH CARE AND THE DEVELOPMENT OF WELFARE STATES

The welfare state is one of the fundamental features in the institutional landscape of modern industrial societies. The development of health care services which seek to protect and promote the health of individuals and communities has been viewed as one of the necessary institutional components of any welfare system. The roots of the contemporary twentieth-century welfare state can be traced back to various important innovations during the second half of the nineteenth century. An example of this kind of innovation in health care was the work of reformers such as Edwin Chadwick in Britain in identifying and documenting the impact of industrialization and urbanization upon the physical environment in which people lived and the health of the population. The 'sanitation reform movement' of the mid-nineteenth century set in train the beginnings of modern public health systems in which action through national or local government institutions sought the achievement of clean water supplies and major improvements in human waste disposal and in housing conditions. The influence of the sanitation movement diffused widely, being felt in both Europe and America. Many of those involved in the sanitation debate in America visited Britain and Europe to exchange ideas and experience. The acceptance of government action to protect the environment and the health of the population was reflected in legislation and the emergence of organizational structures in government from which the institutions of modern health care systems developed. Developments in public health were just part of a broader picture, in which there was an increasing acceptance of

the intervention and growth of government and the application
of knowledge and technology to the social environment.

Individual access to health care in the nineteenth century was
essentially based upon an individual's position in the socio-
economic system. Those who were well-off could afford to pay
for the services of a doctor in their own homes for themselves
and members of their families and households. Other sections
of the population had to rely on joining with others in collective action through groups such as friendly societies to whom
they paid regular contributions with the society contracting
a doctor to provide health care to members. Others sought
care from alternative health care networks provided by family
members, neighbours, healers of various kinds and by taking
drugs or herbal remedies which were purchased from druggists
and chemists. Others relied upon the philanthropic giving of
members of the community which might be organized through
individuals or voluntary groups in order to gain access to health
care. Government involvement in the health care of individuals
for much of the nineteenth century was largely confined to
institutional care in Poor Law institutions or in the provision
of hospitals for the mentally ill and handicapped.

Many commentators on the creation of the welfare state have
linked its evolution to social and political changes associated with
the twin developments of industrialization and capitalism as the
dominant mode of production. Inequality which is inherent to
such an economic structure represents a potential threat to a
stable social and political order. The welfare state initially offered
a restricted set of claims available to a small and visible section
of the community who were most disadvantaged. This system, however, gradually evolved over time into an increasingly
complex and comprehensive method of establishing claims to
resources which may cover the whole population (Flora and
Heidenheimer, 1981b; Gronbjerg, 1977; Marshall, 1965). An
examination of the history of national health care systems in
Britain and America since the nineteenth century demonstrates
this process of extension of government involvement in funding
and service provision to ensure access to health care throughout
the population albeit in very different ways.

In Britain the 1911 National Insurance Act made general
medical services available to manual workers and others on low

incomes and incorporated the principles of social insurance with the individual, the employer and the state making contributions to the cost. Government at both central and local level became increasingly involved in direct provision of health care services during the first half of the twentieth century. The extension of access to health care for the whole population came about through the 1946 National Health Services Act, an Act which has been viewed as a cornerstone of the welfare state in Britain. It provided access for the whole population to hospital care, community-based general medical services and drugs at no direct cost, or at most minimal cost, at the point of receipt of the service. Despite recent changes, such as contracting out some services to private sector providers, organizational changes and growth in private insurance-backed care, the British health care system retains the underlying structure of a universally available service with contributions to its cost from employed individuals, employers and government. The provision of health care services remains a central feature of the British welfare system.

America has often been characterized as being a 'welfare state laggard' and this reluctance to provide access to services has been seen as especially apparent in relation to health care. Important initiatives to extend health care access during the first half of the twentieth century were not initiated by federal or state governments. Professional associations were responsible for the introduction of Blue Cross for hospital care and Blue Shield for general practitioner services in the period following the economic depression of the 1920s and 1930s. Federal government has become more actively involved with the introduction of Medicare and Medicaid in the 1960s and these programmes have meant important changes in access to health care for identifiable sections of the population although falling far short of universal coverage.

In 1983 public expenditure on health care in America represented about 40 per cent of total health care spending in contrast to Britain where almost 89 per cent was financed by government (OECD, 1985a, pp. 12–14). The difference between the two countries was much less marked if the comparison is based on public expenditure relative to GDP which was 5.5 per cent in Britain and 4.5 per cent in America in 1983. It is also important to recognize the considerable growth in public funding of health care in America in recent years. Public financing of health

care in America since the mid-1960s has grown from under
25 per cent of all health care expenditure in 1965 to 40 per
cent in 1983. This substantial increase has occurred during a
period in which there has been a rapid escalation in total health
spending. Historically the role of government in increasing
access to health in America is underestimated by ignoring the
impact of taxation provisions. A very important element in
the extension of health care within the American population
has been contained within the negotiations between employers
and unions since the mid-1940s. Health insurance coverage of
workers and their families has been obtained as part of wage
negotiations and cover purchased from third party insurers. It is
easy to ignore the substantial contribution which tax allowances
to employers and employees have made to the development of
these programmes. As Titmuss (1976) pointed out, we cannot
understand the welfare state without recognizing the manner in
which tax allowances and rebates represent claims to resources
in just the same way as direct payments and services do. The
OECD has estimated tax expenditures on health care in America
to be in excess of $24.2 US billion in 1983 and its inclusion
would increase the total public share of health care spending to
5 per cent of GDP (1985a, p. 27). It is easy to underestimate the
contribution of federal and state governments to ensuring access
to and funding of health care services in American society if the
taxation system is ignored.

HEALTH CARE AND THE ECONOMY

Health care expenditures involve the consumption of a sizeable
proportion of national resources and this use of resources has
grown rapidly in both America and Britain since the Second
World War (see Table 1.1). There has been a similar pattern
of growth in public expenditure on health care during this
period (see Table 1.2). These kinds of estimates of expenditure
are more likely to underestimate rather than overestimate the
true level of spending as they fail to capture fully the entire
range of private expenditures on items such as alternative health
treatments, health care products in nutrition and lifestyle and
over-the-counter patent medicine sales.

Table 1.1 Total health care spending as a percentage of GNP in Britain and America

Year	UK	US
1950	3.9	4.5
1960	3.9	5.3
1970	4.5	7.6
1980	5.8	9.5
1983	6.2	10.8

Sources: Maxwell, 1981; OECD, 1985a.

Table 1.2 Public expenditure on health care as a percentage of GNP in Britain and America

Year	UK	US
1960	3.4	1.3
1965	3.6	1.6
1970	3.9	2.8
1975	5.0	3.7
1980	5.2	4.1
1983	5.5	4.5

Source: OECD, 1985a, p. 12.

Health care spending is not only important in terms of present consumption of resources but also in terms of past and present capital formation within an economy. Both private and public providers of health care services have made major investments in plant and equipment and in a wide range of facilities such as hospitals, health centres and general practice and these kinds of facilities utilize valuable land assets, especially in urban areas. Historically the producers of pharmaceutical and medical equipment have also made substantial capital investment in processing plant.

Whilst health care does entail considerable capital investment it is also a relatively labour intensive industry and the growth of health care within the economies of developed industrialized countries is reflected in changes in employment structures. Routh (1980) has estimated that professional and semi-professional employment in Britain's health industry increased from 170,000 in 1921 to 601,000 in 1971. The proportion of health care workers in the total labour force also grew from 0.9

per cent in 1921 to 2.4 per cent in 1971. If all workers engaged in providing services to the health care industry such as transport, cleaning, catering, laundering, reception services and so on were included then the substantial and growing utilization of labour in health care would be even more obvious. The inclusion of these service workers would still represent an underestimate as it would not include those employed in the manufacture of products for use in health care, especially pharmaceuticals, and those who provide services such as publicity and public relations to health providers.

The economic importance of health stretches beyond national boundaries in an activity such as pharmaceutical production and distribution. Large multinational pharmaceutical companies are now well established and their activities extend throughout the international economy. This development appears to be spreading beyond pharmaceuticals and into the mainstream of health service provision as large private health care providers begin to market their services into other countries as is demonstrated by a growing American presence in the British health care market.

TECHNOLOGY AND SOCIAL SERVICE PRODUCTION

There is no doubt that health care occupies an important position both in the structure of welfare states in industrialized countries and as a major industry in these economies. It is surprising therefore that little attempt has been made to apply knowledge and ideas derived from the study of technological change in manufacturing and service industries elsewhere in an economy to the study of the health care industry and indeed the welfare state in general.

An important assumption in this book is that technology and technological change cannot be seen as events which occur completely separately from the generation of goods and services in the welfare system. Present theories of the welfare state tend to constrict the role of technology to its impact on economic growth which is then viewed as determining the availability of resources for distribution through social service programmes in the welfare state. This position ignores the fact that a major industry such as health care has an identifiable technological base which is used to produce a range of products and services. If we hope to understand the development of social services such as health, and welfare states in general, then we must examine the technological base of production within the welfare state. In addition we must study how this technology changes over time and how it is both influenced by, and in turn influences, other areas of production within an economy.

The literature on technological change casts light on critical questions such as:

- what is technology?
- how are inventions translated into new product and process technologies?
- what factors influence the adoption of new technologies?
- is technological change affected by the social context in which it takes place?
- what is the role of social invention and innovation?

If these questions are addressed in relation to social services such as health care then an important new dimension can be added to our present theories of welfare state development.

The remainder of this chapter briefly summarizes selected aspects of the available literature on technological change which will then be used to develop a framework for analysing technological change in health care in the subsequent chapters of Part I. Any readers already familiar with this literature may prefer to proceed to the development and application of these ideas to health care production in Chapter 2.

What is technology?

Considering the vast literature on technology and technological change, there are relatively few writers who attempt to define and conceptualize what is meant by the term 'technology'. The definition which has been adopted here is drawn from the work of Gehlen (1980) in which technology is broadly conceived as either a substitute for, or an enhancement of, biological human functioning. Gehlen says that technologies can be classified into three major categories.

The first are those which replace human organs and may perform beyond the capacity of those organs, such as robots in car assembly-line tasks or plastic hip replacement joints in the human body. The second are those which enhance our bodily functions, such as hand tools like screwdrivers or hammers, household equipment like vacuum cleaners or food processors and communication technologies like the telephone or electronic mail facilities. The third are those technologies which facilitate human functioning by relieving or disengaging human organs, such as forms of human transportation like cars or the analysis of complex information by computer. If human functioning is taken to incorporate emotional functioning, as well as bodily functioning, then this definition of technology is appropriate to a consideration of technology in social service production including health care.

Gehlen notes that whilst the links between experimental science and technology constitute the foundation of industrial organization, the effects of change are also apparent in the social, political and personal realms of human activity. Technology is more than the application of scientific and other knowledge through machines to identifiable tasks. Tasks are performed in organizations which consist of people and which generate products and services intended for consumption by people. Changes in social and cultural organization create an environment which influences the substance, direction and rate of technical change (Pacey, 1983, p. 6). It is not possible to understand technology without incorporating this social dimension into the analysis. This point is of special importance in an analysis of health care technology because health care straddles the boundaries between the industrial, social, political and personal aspects of human life.

How does technology change over time?

Much of our knowledge about technological change comes from the study of how technological change contributes both to the production of goods and services in an economy and to economic development in general. Most writers make a distinction between the generation of knowledge on the one hand, and its application to the production of goods and services on the other. This distinction has been expressed in a variety of ways, such as science and technology (Jewkes *et. al.*, 1969), basic research and development work (Freeman, 1982), fundamental science and innovation (van Duijn, 1983) and invention and innovation (Mensch, 1979). A second distinction is made between innovations themselves and the way in which those innovations spread within industries, between industries and between countries. The spread of innovations amongst potential adopters is frequently termed diffusion. Invention, innovation and diffusion will now be discussed in greater detail. However it is important to recognize that whilst the distinctions between these three components do provide a useful framework for analysis and discussion it would be wrong to see them as discrete and defined phases in a simple sequential model of change. In practice there may be considerable overlapping and discontinuities between these phases and complex feedback effects between different parts in the change process.

Invention

Important inventions are popularly equated with the actions of particular individuals – radio with Marconi, penicillin with Fleming, the jet engine with Whittle and so on. Ruttan (1959, p. 601) describes this as the 'transcendentalist' approach in which the record of invention is a description of the work of individual genius which occurs in a mostly unpredictable manner. Invention is seemingly disconnected from the flow of ideas which have preceded the 'great discovery' and is accordingly seen as representing a major break with the past.

An alternative approach is to see invention as an element in a continuous evolutionary process in which it is market demand from consumers and producers which elicits the necessary inventions. The phrase 'necessity is the mother of invention' encapsulates this view and confines the role of the individual inventor to being a minor actor in the process of change. As will be explained later this approach to an understanding of invention has been subsequently transferred into accounts of innovation. There are limitations in this type of single-factor approach to explaining social changes such as those generated by invention. Raymond Boudon (1986, chapter 6) has warned of the dangers of seeing social change as solely a demand-led process in which the resultant changes are seen as the 'natural' consequences of demand-based factors. Incorrect interpretations of change based solely upon demand factors are encouraged by three temptations: first, the temptation to generalize from those changes that are a response to demand to all changes, second, the temptation to explain what is happening now by what has happened in the past and third, the temptation to see change as a functional requirement of a closed system.

A third approach to understanding invention derives from the work of Usher (1954) who presents invention as a process in which a wide range of ideas, material things and human behaviour are brought together in new ways. Individuals may provide a major contribution through acts of insight which help to overcome problems rather like a 'key' piece in a jigsaw. However, these acts of insight are of varying degrees of importance in a 'cumulative synthesis' (Usher, 1954, p. 60) through which a full realization of a new picture or pattern gradually becomes apparent and subsequently realized. Watson's (1981) description of his discovery, with Crick, of the shape of the DNA molecule vividly illustrates this process of continual knowledge building combined with an act of insight which orders knowledge in a new way.

The role of a single individual or research group in science and invention was questioned by Merton (Mulkay, 1972, p. 18) who pointed out the frequency of multiple identification of the same scientific discoveries by various individuals and groups who seemingly acted independently from each other. 'Multiple discoveries' are often accompanied by public conflict as to who was the first to have achieved the discovery. As Mulkay (1972, p. 18) concludes, multiple discoveries may not be the predominant form of invention, but they do occur sufficiently frequently to cast doubt on the notion that invvention represents a radical break with existing knowledge.

Usher suggested that there are four steps in invention; the first involves the recognition of the problem, the second the assembly and manipulation of available information, the third entails acts of individual insight in which new relations between ideas are established and the fourth a process of critical revision in which understanding of this new pattern becomes more fully understood and its application explored through further acts of insight. It is not, however, possible to predict in advance what will be the substance of these acts of invention nor their timing.

Innovation

Most writers seek to distinguish between invention and innovation. Invention is part of the generation of new ideas and materials through advances in fundamental science whilst innovation entails the application of such ideas to the production of goods and services. Invention does not necessarily lead to innovation and often there may be a substantial time lag between invention and innovation. In Usher's terms further acts of 'cumulative synthesis' are usually required before the relevance of new knowledge and inventions is understood and the technical means found to translate them into the production of goods and services. There is, for example, a substantial amount of development work required after the identification of a new pharmaceutical drug and before its use to treat illness in the community. A method has to be established for isolating the drug in a stable form, the clinical effectiveness and safety of the drug must be demonstrated and a method devised for achieving large scale production and marketing. The time lags involved in this development work are well illustrated by the history of penicillin. The isolation of penicillin by Fleming in 1929 did not of itself establish either a method of stabilizing the drug nor of showing its clinical potential. It was a decade before Florey and Chain were able to achieve these goals and a further time period elapsed before, with the application of substantial research funding from America, large-scale production of penicillin became a reality.

Mensch (1979) argues that there are definite qualitative differences in innovations and that it is possible to identify those innovations which represent a radical change from existing technologies. He describes these differences by use of an analogy with what he refers to as an evolutionary tree in which 'Every fork in a branch stands for the opening of a new path – a new method of operation or a new technology' (p. 47). He refers to these departures from existing practices as 'basic innovations' in which new products and processes are translated into new markets and industrial branches. Mensch's conception of basic innovations is similar to Boudon's (1986) view of mutation innovations as opposed to demand innovations in that they entail a break with the past and generate major structural changes. Once the initial product or service is produced, there commonly follows a series of 'improvement innovations' in which the product or service is developed and its full potential realized. A flow of related products may also emerge with innovations across several areas of production interacting with each other and generating further improvements. These improvement innovations are similar to Boudon's notion of demand innovations in that they help to realize fully the benefits of basic innovations and the broad structural arrangements that have emerged alongside these innovations. The development of television vividly demonstrates the flow of improvement innovations. There have beenn changes in the size of television receivers from large, heavy, valve-based sets with monochrome pictures to the contemporary colour receivers with immense choice in size from hand-held miniaturized sets to very large public arena sets. Television has also become linked to a flow of related products such as video recorders, video cameras and audio systems. The earlier example of penicillin also illustrates this process of improvement innovation. The initial production of penicillin for civilian use began in 1945. From 1947 to 1951 many improvements in the product were made including the introduction of penicillin-based drugs such as chlorotetracycline and tetracycline. In the late 1950s and 1960s the isolation of the peniccillin nucleus led to the production of a new grouping of semi-synthetic penicillin-related drugs such as Penbritin.

There seems to be broad agreement that there are limits to the improvements that can be made to a single product. As Boulding explains: 'No growth process is exponential for very long. All of them follow what are called logistic curves with eventually diminishing rates of growth' (1981, p. 144). Examination of the development of any major innovation over time is likely to reveal an 'S' curve showing the gradual slowing in the rate of improvement innovations after the initial basic service or product innovation. A comparison of the histories of a range of products will however show wide variations in the specific shape of the 'S' curve.

Diffusion

Once an innovation is capable of being used in production, what factors influence the adoption of innovations and the diffusion of innovations among potential users in a particular industry, between industries and between different countries? Rogers defines diffusion as 'the process by which an innovation is communicated through certain channels over time among the members of a social system . . . concerned with new ideas' (1983, p. 5). Writers about diffusion identify two main approaches to explaining the diffusion process. The first approach emphasizes the importance of learning both by having the innovation explained and demonstrated and by practical experience of the innovation. The second approach uses the idea of 'disease' in which an innovation is transmitted by 'carriers' and other mechanisms and 'caught' by individual units who are susceptible to contagion.

In their study of industrialization and diffusion Kenwood and Lougheed (1982) summarize the factors which they believe influence diffusion and similar factors have been identified elsewhere in the literature.

1   Demand – what will be the market for the new product or service that will be produced or for an existing product if it is produced through a new process innovation?
2   Capital – what will be the capital requirements for realizing an innovation?
3   Natural resources – does the innovation require particular natural resources and are these available, accessible and sustainable?
4   Labour – is the supply of labour of the necessary quality as well as quantity and what will be the cost of that labour?
5   Technological factors – how do potential adopters perceive the innovation in terms of its technological advantages? Rogers (1983, pp. 15–16) has argued that there are five aspects which influence this perception. First they must be convinced that the innovation is better than the current

product, process or service; second that it fits in with the traditions, needs and values of the potential adopters' organization; third that the innovation is not so complex that it is difficult to understand and therefore to disseminate within the organization and to consumers; fourth that the possibility exists of being able to test the innovation on a limited scale before fully committing investment capital; fifth that the innovation is visible, both within the organization and outside it to consumers and competitors.

6   Scale – some innovations involve large scale change either in their own right or as parts of technological clusters of related innovations. The capital, labour and organizational demands of an innovation may be beyond the scope of potential adopters to manage. Action may therefore require a number of groups to act together to generate the various elements in the innovation.

7   Infrastructure – innovations may be dependent upon the successful adoption of other innovations before they become viable; for instance, marketing strategy based upon telephone canvassing requires the existence of a widely disseminated infrastructure of home telephones and the home video industry depends not only on households purchasing video recorders but also the prior existence of an extensive infrastructure of television ownership. The capital requirements of establishing a new infrastructure and discontinuing an existing one may provide formidable barriers to an innovation. Many conservationists, for example, would argue that maintaining the petrol engine as the basic technology of our personal transport system in the motor car is a reflection more of the capital cost of replacing the present infrastructure of car manufacturing than of the limitations of technological innovation.

8   Language – language is an important factor in the communication of an innovation amongst potential adopters. Barriers to diffusion may come from the technical language surrounding an innovation as well as language barriers between and within countries.

9   Culture – the values and norms associated with particular cultures will influence both the decision to adopt and the speed of diffusion.

Much of the analysis of diffusion of radical technologies in both new products and new production processes has come from the work of economists. The research work of Edwin Mansfield (1969, 1977) and his colleagues over many years has greatly contributed to our understanding of innovation within economic structures and his work has influenced many other researchers. The emphasis on innovations in manufacturing leads to a focus on how an innovation will affect the factors of production, namely labour and capital, and how these changes will subsequently affect the quantity, quality and speed of production. The influence of changes in production upon cost structures, and therefore the profitability of manufacturing, has also been a research focus. There is broad agreement about factors which influence both the decision to adopt and the speed of adoption (Freeman, 1982; Kenwood and Lougheed, 1982; Mansfield, 1969 and 1977; Ray, 1984; Rogers, 1983; Scherer, 1984; Stoneman, 1983).

The first of the two main factors is profitability. Is there an economic advantage in adopting the innovation? Will profitability be enhanced and does the rate of return compare favourably with other investment options? To what extent is, or can, the innovation be protected through patents or licensing arrangements? Is the innovation likely to be profitable for the firm supplying the innovator firm as well as for the innovator? The second main factor is capital investment. What is the size of capital investment required relative to the profitability and current asset base of the enterprise? Does the enterprise have access to capital to pursue the innovation?

There is recognition of other factors in the economic literature, despite the primary focus on profitability and capital requirements. The complexity of the innovation will affect the learning demands placed upon the labour force within an organization, and with some innovations this will extend to the end user. The more complex the innovation the greater the barrier to adoption and to the speed of diffusion. The attitudes of management have also been seen as important both in their willingness to take risks, and in the extensiveness of networks within their own industry and other industries. The more outgoing and cosmopolitan the management the more likely they are to innovate and to be amongst the leaders of an innovation.

Rogers (1983, pp. 245–51) has put forward a method of classifying adopters according to the speed at which they adopt an innovation. He argues that if an examination of adoption amongst a population of potential adopters is made, adoption will follow the pattern of a normal distribution and five categories of adopters are identifiable according to their position in the distribution. The first innovators are adventurous, have an extensive network of relations and have the resources necessary to take risks. Early adopters are well integrated in their geographical or industrial community and are opinion leaders in these groups. The early majority decide to adopt ideas just before the average member of the social system and they are followers rather than leaders. The late majority are likely to have been initially sceptical about the innovation but adopt in response to economic pressures and the pressure of opinion as the level of adoption has built up. The laggards are the final group to adopt and tend to be very traditional and rather isolated and localized in their outlook.

Ray (1984, pp. 81–2) has examined the diffusion of a number of major industrial processes, like steelmaking and machine tools. He concludes that diffusion of a process innovation between companies in different countries takes about four or five years, but that it takes about twenty years for the innovation to be totally diffused throughout an industry. He indicates that diffusion takes much longer when the capital requirements of the innovation are relatively low. This finding indicates that service innovations, including those in social service production which tend to be labour rather than capital intensive, may have longer diffusion time spans than product innovations. This could be a reflection of learning and communication barriers to rapid diffusion of new labour technologies.

Technological change and its social context

The analysis of technological change and the relationship of those changes to economic development has been carried out predominantly by economists and economic historians. The explanations which they offer emphasize the requirements of the economic market place. Factors such as profit maximization, capital availability, labour supply and cost, consumer demand

and macro-economic cycles have been presented as the main variables to be considered. There is, however, some recognition of the influence of individual actors, especially the behaviour of entrepreneurs in assessing risks before deciding whether to pursue the implementation of an innovation. The fact that innovations may have major social consequences is occasionally recognized within the discussion. However, the relationship between technological change in the economic system and social change is commonly presented in a hierarchical manner in which economic changes are seen as determining the direction of social changes.

Technological change does not occur in isolation from social and political life. Invention, innovation and diffusion take place over a long period of time and involve individuals, work groups and wider organizational structures. In any organization or group of organizations the structures, communication systems, values and cultures of the organizations and individuals within them influence the direction and acceptance of technological change.

Four illustrations of the way in which the social context may have an impact upon technological change will now be briefly described.

1 *Attitudes to science and technology within the scientific community* The importance of social influences has been well documented in explanations of scientific discovery. An analysis of what problems are regarded as being important to study, how they are to be studied and which projects will be supported by research funding suggests that there is strong pressure to conform to socially accepted patterns of understanding and action (Mulkay, 1972, pp. 18–19). As Miller (1978) observes: 'Everyone approaches the world with ontological assumptions, confident presuppositions about what is there' (p. 224). There are many instances where important observations have been made but their significance has not been recognized because the existing framework of theoretical knowledge has not allowed the meaning of these observations to become apparent to the observer. An example of this phenomenon is given by Hawkins (1988, p. 42) who notes that the notion that the universe was expanding could have been predicted on the basis of Newton's

theory of gravity at any time from the late seventeenth century. The fact that it was not is attributable to the firm belief that the existence of a static universe was a 'given' around which all other relevant knowledge must be organized and interpreted. If observations do not fit with a strongly established theory they are likely to be discredited, or *ad hoc* changes made to the theory to try to accommodate them. The critical feature is that the theoretical framework available at any one point in time is at least in part socially constructed and maintained.

Mulkay (1972) suggests that there are three main reasons why the direction and process of scientific discovery is moulded in this way. First, scientists, including social scientists, are socialized in an education system which seeks to convey an established body of knowledge and accepted means of furthering that knowledge. Second, most professional research communities, whilst espousing individual autonomy, display a trend towards authoritarian structures in which membership and rewards are based upon acceptance of existing research paradigms. This trend is demonstrated in the increasing use of research teams in which each member has a specialized role and which often leads to the creation of management structures in which a high degree of centralized control and coordination is evident. Third, professional recognition is partly based upon the presentation and sharing of information. Ideas and research methodologies which fall outside the existing paradigms in relation to a particular problem risk both the rejection of the ideas themselves and of those who advocate them, and their adoption is likely to be viewed negatively within the research community. The emphasis on sharing information also means that there is a continual flow of material which conforms, within certain parameters, to what is currently accepted thinking. Scientific discovery and invention is therefore subject to considerable social influence through the education of scientists, the organization of scientific work and influences on scientists in terms of personal and collective recognition.

2   The influence of organizational and management structures   Technological change can take place in the system of social organization itself, an event which Mensch (1979, chapter 2) has described as a 'nontechnical basic innovation'. This view has been mirrored in the work of several other writers. Schumpeter (Freeman, 1982, pp. 216–17) acknowledged that organizational and managerial innovations are often of equal importance to innovations in products and processes. Boulding (1981) has described the existence of a dynamic relationship between technical and non-technical basic innovations in which it must be recognized that innovations in either sphere can create opportunities for innovations in the other. Adopting this stance means that major innovations in social service organizations should not be seen as solely technical events, but can also reflect major changes in social and political organization and these changes can in turn feed back into other production technologies.

Hummon (1984) points out that invention and innovation in modern industrialized economies are complex activities which usually require formal organizations to sustain them over the substantial time periods which are needed to realize an innovation. Innovations in how those organizations operate are important both as a consequence of product innovation and as a catalyst to ongoing product innovation. Hummon uses Arthur Stinchcombe's work on organizational form to emphasize the importance of features such as organizational size, training and communication structures, task organization and the differentiation of tasks which is apparent in the division of labour. The more sophisticated the general technological environment then the more detailed the division of labour is likely to be, and there will be the increasing growth of professional management structures which control the planning and implementation of technological change (Montgomery, 1979).

The influence of the organizational and managerial environment can operate at many different levels. Wallace (1982) has described the impact of both the social organization within and outside an industry in the development of coal mining and iron and ordinance manufacture from 1600 to 1900. He points out that the development of new ideas and their application always involves a work group within an organization that has been in existence for a considerable period of time, working on the basic ideas before they are realized. The lifespan of the work group is also linked to the life of the total organization, with successful innovation being more likely in organizations that have survived for two or more generations. Survival is seen as facilitating the accumulation and analysis of relevant information. Innovation also depends upon the perception of innovation within the total organization. It is promoted by a climate which supports innovation and regards the commitment of funds from the enterprise as a necessary component of an investment strategy. Wallace (1982, p. 153) also identifies two important influences within the wider social environment which affect innovation. The first he asserts concerns relative public perceptions of scientific knowledge on the one hand and technology on the other. Public support for technology rather than scientific knowledge as the major contributor to social progress will tend to encourage innovation. The second influence is the effect of social mobility which may be critical to innovation by encouraging communication networks between creative people in the middle and lower classes and in creating incentives to acquire wealth, property and social progress. Linkages between members of the upper classes and other members of society may also be important in encouraging dialogue about how to solve technical problems.

3 *The social organization of labour* The social organization of labour (rather than just the supply and cost of labour) may influence, and be influenced by, technological change. Blackburn *et al.* (1985, p. 9) observe that technological innovations in products and processes have major implications for the labour market, but that changes are influenced by the attitudes and structures of organized labour and wider social attitudes toward unemployment, job mobility and retraining. Benson and Lloyd (1983) have asserted that the structure and development of labour movements has been influenced by long-term cycles or Kondratieff waves in the international economy in which the position of some groups of workers in the labour market is undermined by technological changes during each cycle. The impact of steam power on textile factories in the first Kondratieff wave during the early nineteenth century undermined the position of weavers and stockingers and saw the emergence of craft unions and collective bargaining at the local level. Innovations in communication and transport technologies in the second Kondratieff during the second half of the nineteenth century were influential in increasing urbanization and attempts to introduce mass production techniques. It is this period which saw the formation of

national unions and independent working-class political parties. The third Kondratieff in the first half of the twentieth century depended upon science-based industries and the factory production line. Centralized bargaining between labour organizations and producer organizations became regulated by extensive state regulation and coercion. The beginning of the fourth Kondratieff wave in the 1970s and 1980s is seen by Benson and Lloyd as being characterized by a sustained attack on the ability of unions to control the levels of machine manning in the production line. The general proposition that each wave of technological innovation has influenced the development of organized labour, which has in turn influenced the realization of innovations, supports the more general proposition that technological change both creates opportunities for innovations in social life and that these innovations create further opportunities for technological change. The links between technological change in health care and long wave economic cycles will be examined in more detail in Chapter 5.

4 The role of government The influence which perceptions of science and technology within national and international communities might have upon the speed and acceptance of technological change was noted earlier. Government plays an important role in both reflecting public attitudes through its policies towards science and technology and also in influencing those perceptions in the manner it portrays technological change to the general community. The very substantial contribution which many national governments make towards research and development in the private sector has already been noted but governments also directly fund research in government establishments and universities and other tertiary institutions. Governments also commonly take a more direct responsibility for provision of certain goods and services, including social services, and this responsibility also entails research and development spending to promote technological change in these activities. Mansfield (1969, p. 165) estimated that in the mid-1960s the American Health, Education and Welfare Department was spending about 13 per cent of its total expenditure on research and development with about one-third on basic research and two-thirds on applied research.

Capital and labour both influence technological change and government policies greatly affect the availability and quality of the factors of production. The environment for business investment is affected by a wide range of measures adopted by governments which encourage or discourage investment. Depreciation allowances, subsidies, subsidized loans, location and relocation incentives, import controls are just a few of the range of instruments that are used to make an impact on decisions about investment. The provision of capital through private savings is also susceptible to a similar range of incentives and disincentives. Where goods and services are provided directly by government, or through direct funding of other providers, then government is directly involved in making capital investment decisions. Just as government is a powerful influence upon capital it also plays a critical role in the labour market. Technological change in industrial countries has made knowledge and information analysis central to economic development. In this type of 'information economy' (Stonier, 1983, pp. 12–13) education is of pivotal importance and government usually plays a central role both in determining the overall educational framework and as a provider of education services. Government also prescribes the general conditions under which labour is employed through measures such as minimum wage, sick pay, holidays, equal employment opportunity and many other legislative measures. In addition government is directly and indirectly a major employer in industrialized countries and in this role as employer has considerable impact upon the labour market.

As many writers on technological change observe there is no technological change which does not generate costs beyond those narrowly defined within product or process development. As has already been noted, where radical innovations are involved there are significant impacts upon the labour force and the organization of labour. Many changes entail extensive retraining of labour and displacement through redundancies. Industrial countries recognize the costs of unemployment through income support payments to the unemployed. There is also recognition that there are health costs associated with loss of employment. In addition to labour costs there are capital costs such as the impact of technological change upon the natural resource environment and the future viability of existing plant and equipment. Government plays an important role in determining what the costs of technological change are and who will bear those costs. Government action may vary widely from allowing the costs to lie wherever they fall to determining who will pay and how much. Government provision of social services in particular often involves an implicit acceptance by government that the costs of technological change should be borne by the community as a whole through publicly financed and provided social services rather than being borne by particular individuals and their families.

Social invention and innovation

The earlier discussion of technological change was based almost entirely upon consideration of innovation in products or the processes by which those products are made. The way in which the social context influences technological innovations has been described above but the possibility of innovation occurring in the system of social organization itself and subsequently affecting technological change must also be acknowledged.

Brooks (1982) has described social invention as new ways of organizing social systems and relationships and it involves a similar process of cumulative insight as that described for other forms of technological change. Social innovation is the process by which these inventions are realized in new social relationships. Just as all technological innovations are influenced by their social environment so social inventions are influenced by the environment of the physical technology in which they occur. Social innovation may involve a radical change in the technological base or improvements upon existing technology in the same way as technical innovations. Brooks outlines a continuum for inventions and innovations reflecting the relative importance of social and technological factors. He believes that there are some inventions which are almost entirely technical, especially where new materials are involved. However, the realization of these inventions involves auxiliary technologies where social invention and innovation may play a part. There are social inventions and innovations such as health mainte- nance organizations or negative income taxation where the changes define new social relationships which may subsequently incorporate physical technologies to help realize the full value of that social innovation. Brooks also recognizes the idea of clusters of innovations in which a core innovation, such as the car or telephone, becomes linked to a wide range of both technical and social innovations in order to extract the full value from those innovations. He refers to these as sociotechnical inventions and innovations.

Brooks (1982, pp. 10–24) classifies social inventions and innovations into four categories:

1 Marketing inventions and innovations – new ways of marketing services and products to enable market penetration and maintenance.
2 Managerial inventions and innovations – changes which occur within the organization of private companies or public bureaucracies which increase the level of productivity or the quality of products and services.
3 Political inventions and innovations – changes in legislation or other elements of government policy which incorporate new structures or mechanisms for achieving government policy goals.
4 Institutional inventions or innovations – the creation of new institutional arrangements in order to provide new services or products. These changes may occur at the local level in response to local factors in the social and technical environment.

This classification is a valuable one and will later be incorporated into the conceptualization of technological innovation in health care with some modification. The distinction between managerial and institutional changes does not recognize that both forms can have a 'macro' and 'micro' dimension. Managerial changes may be related to a specific plant or localized organization and institutional changes, say in the public sector, may be on a national level. It seems better to combine these two types of social invention and innovation and recognize that they may involve structural changes which transform the institutional environment within which the service or product is produced as well as much broader changes in the management of the process.

2 Technological Change and Health Care

HEALTH CARE: DEFINING THE TECHNOLOGICAL BASE OF A SOCIAL SERVICE

There is a wealth of material in the medical literature describing the history of advances in medical technology. Much of this writing concerns quite specific innovations, for instance in the development of a vaccine against a particular disease, or the development of a distinct surgical technique. Alternatively writers focus upon the deeds of famous figures in scientific or medical practice. The interest being expressed in technology is essentially secondary to the dominant interest in a disease or the exploits of a famous person. Usually the term technology is either not clearly defined or defined in an arbitrary manner. This general approach to the role of technology in health care has been well demonstrated in the contemporary debate concerning the role which technological innovations may have played in the rapid escalation of health care expenditure in industrially developed countries, especially during the 1960s and 1970s. Altman and Wallack (1979) observe that few studies of the role of technology on health expenditure levels actually attempt to define what they mean by health care technology. The majority of studies in effect treat technology as what is left over after accounting for all other forms of expenditure.

The public perception of health in contemporary society is most probably of a complex activity which is beyond the comprehension of all but a few *cognoscenti*. The linkage between health and scientific endeavour is established in the public perception through the vast array of machines and instruments which attend all levels of medical care. An emphasis upon the tools, machines and procedures of medical care technology in Western societies has been explained in terms of the association between medical and physical sciences in Western culture. Osherson and AmaraSingham have pointed to the growing emphasis in science, since the eighteenth century, upon empirical observation and explanations based on physical causation. Those at the forefront of generating knowledge through empirical science were also frequently interested and involved in developing knowledge about the functioning of the body and disease. Miller (1978) has described how an understanding of the physical world, and machines in particular, helped develop our understanding of how the body works through the extensive use of analogies with the mechanical world.

It is this notion of the body as a machine which Osherson and AmaraSingham have explored in detail, demonstrating how this idea linked medicine to the wider social and cultural milieu in Western societies. The human body produced labour as part of the total industrial machine. Machines could be maintained, repaired, developed and replaced through the generation and application of scientific knowledge and technology. By analogy the potential was seen to exist for the human body to be serviced as medical science increased our understanding of bodily functioning and complementary technologies were generated which would enable bodily functioning to be maintained and enhanced. The 'glamour' medical technologies of contemporary society, such as organ transplantation and new birth technologies, are obvious manifestations of this mechanistic ideal which is still apparent as we approach the end of the twentieth century. Gehlen's definition of technology, which was described in Chapter 1, reflects a similar view that machines and the human body are intrinsically linked by defining technology in terms of the impact of physical machines upon the functioning of the human machine.

Osherson and AmaraSingham have outlined the transformation in the relationship between doctor and patient during the nineteenth century. Initially the doctor was dependent on the information provided by the patient in the course of person to person discussion. Both doctor and patient had an active part to play in the determination of diagnosis and treatment. The gradual adoption of diagnostic techniques and tools, which were used by the doctor on the body of the patient, changed not only the information base of diagnosis but also the position of the patient who became predominantly a passive spectator to the actions of the doctor. The transformation in the relationship between doctor and patient reflects a perception of disease and illness in which symptoms of ill health are regarded as evidence of a defect in the mechanical world of the body which has to be identified and repaired. Osherson and AmaraSingham demonstrate how this mechanistic view has had a widespread impact on health care not only in the doctor–patient relationship but also in the training of doctors, the development of medical intervention techniques, the medical control over childbirth and in the attitudes toward death and its management in medical institutions in Western societies.

Foucault (Armstrong, 1983), like Osherson and Amara-Singham, has described the growth in medical knowledge and technology during the nineteenth century as the development of 'the reading of the body' of the individual patient. Armstrong (1983, pp. 8–9) has extended this analysis, using the example of the Edinburgh Dispensary for TB patients at the end of the nineteenth century and the beginning of the twentieth century, to describe how the conception of illness included the recognition that health was not just something which existed within the hospital walls but also extended into the community. Disease existed not just in the one body but in the 'spaces between people'. The acceptance of the potential power of medical knowledge held out the possibility that knowledge of the individual body might yield an understanding of the 'social body'. Professional knowledge of the social body derived by the medical and social sciences could then be used to monitor and modify the functioning of the social body and counteract the effects of social problems and disruption caused by social and economic changes. The potential capacity to engineer a social order, in which group functioning, as well as individual functioning, might be maintained and enhanced, flowed from this organic view of society.

These changes in the construction of medical knowledge and its application did not occur in isolation from economic, social and political changes. The central thesis of Osherson and AmaraSingham's work is that medicine is both influenced by and in turn influences the cultural environment in any society. The growth in health care systems and health care professions which lay claim to be able to maintain, and indeed in the future perfect, the human machine both individually and collectively can be viewed as playing an intrinsic role in the development of industrial society. These changes reflect perceived links between science, technology and a dynamic economic system which create opportunities for human progress and which will be discussed in more detail later in this book.

CLASSIFYING HEALTH CARE TECHNOLOGIES

Is it possible to classify the range of technologies used in health care? In Chapter 1 Gehlen's (1980) definition of technology was adopted which emphasized technology as enhancing or substituting for biological functioning. This definition was subsequently extended to include emotional and social functioning. This general approach to technology seems appropriate to health care acknowledging that some technologies affect the functioning of the consumer of health care directly whilst others influence the capacities of those providing health care services to consumers. What constitutes 'progress' and 'betterment' for the individual and the 'social' body can be seen as closely related because the threat of illness, disease and infirmity may affect many people, not just the individual.

Any attempt to conceptualize technology in medical care must be able to encompass the social dimensions of that technology rather than narrowly perceiving medical technology solely in terms of machines and technical procedures which are applied to individuals. The examination of the literature on technological change in Chapter 1 pointed to the limitations of seeing change solely as modifications to a set of products and services and the manner in which they are produced. The social environment in which technology exists and is modified influences the innovations which are adopted and how they are adopted. The social environment itself has a technological base which is both modified by innovations in the production of goods and services and which in turn generates technological changes which create new opportunities for innovation in goods and services. Within this broad definition of technology it is then possible to identify specific types of health technology including 'non-technical' or 'social' technologies.

The following classification draws upon the literature reviewed in the initial chapter and the work of a number of writers on health care and social innovation, especially Birenbaum (1981), Brooks (1982), Sidel (1971) and Stoman (1976).

Diagnostic technologies

Diagnostic technologies allow the functioning of the body to be monitored and assessed and the presence of disease to be diagnosed. The development of a simple tool such as the stethoscope made an important contribution to the ability of doctors to obtain direct information about the functioning of the body. The range of diagnostic technologies has become more complex and more extensive with the introduction of innovations in mechanical technologies such as the microscope, X-rays, electrocardiogram and CAT scanners. Alongside these innovations has been the growth in knowledge about the chemical properties of the human body and corresponding technologies to monitor these characteristics.

Treatment technologies

These are technologies which enable interventions to be made which modify the effects of disease and disability. These interventions may enable a patient to return to the level of functioning prior to the onset of the disease or disabling condition, or they may improve or allow the maintenance of a level of functioning which would not have been possible without the intervention, or they may facilitate a level of functioning previously unattainable for that individual. Treatment technologies can range from surgery, drug therapy, organ replacement or maintenance to physiotherapy, acupuncture and 'alternative' treatments of many kinds. Frequently treatments are combined in a total intervention package and in the case of surgical interventions they are dependent on a variety of supporting technologies such as anaesthesia, antisepsis and blood transfusion.

Disease prevention and health maintenance technologies

These technologies cover both those aimed at the health of individuals and those which influence the health care of large groups or total populations. There are numerous individual technologies which would come in this category including:

- immunization programmes which seek to prevent the incidence of specific diseases;
- programmes of exercise and nutritional programmes aimed at combating disease or promoting good health;
- pre- and post-natal care programmes which aim to promote the health of mother, baby and family;
- general health education programmes which may seek to control specific conditions such as alcohol and general drug abuse or prevent the spread of disease.

Historically measures to modify the general environment in which people live have played an important part in influencing the level of health within large populations. Public health programmes to ensure a clean water supply, adequate sanitation, industrial and road safety and good standards of housing are obvious examples of such innovations. These technologies frequently drew upon technologies derived elsewhere within society especially in mechanical and civil engineering.

Health organization and delivery technologies

Using Brooks' work on social invention and innovation it is clear that changes in the way in which health care has been organized and delivered constitute an important component in technological innovation in health care and therefore in the total technological base of health care. In the previous chapter a distinction was made between three main elements in this area of health technology, namely management/institutional technology, political technology and marketing technology. Changes in the way services have been organized and the institutional frameworks within which they operate have to be assessed if the development of health care is to be understood – for example, in accounting for the changing role of the hospital during the nineteenth and twentieth centuries. Similarly the movement towards increasing centralization of services and the growth of health care specialization have to be viewed as important examples of technological innovation that have had a substantial impact on the evolution of health care. As has already been observed, governments at central and local level have played a part in determining the pattern of health care services in economically developed societies. Decisions by governments about the organizational and financial basis upon which health care is to be produced and consumed represent crucial sources of technological change.

The end use of health care technology

An analysis of health care technology must take into account the distinctions between final and intermediate services and marketed and non-marketed services as identified by Gershuny (1983a). Health care products and services are provided sometimes directly to final consumers and sometimes indirectly through producers of other health care services. Decisions about what will be consumed and by whom are part of the organizational technology of health care which must be considered when seeking to understand the complete picture of technological change in the production of goods and services within a health care system.

Health care technology generates a complex flow of both goods and services in which there may be several users of health care outputs. Some products, such as pharmaceutical drugs, are consumed directly by people who either buy them from a chemist or have them prescribed by doctors. However, some drugs, and a wide range of diagnostic and treatment equipment, are actually consumed by health care workers. These products are frequently being used by one group of health care workers to provide services to another group, thereby assisting these workers in providing a service to consumers. Workers in the health care industry frequently add intermediate services in the flow from production to consumption; for example, a doctor's prescription for a pharmaceutical drug follows an appointment and assessment of the consumer's condition and the consumption of the drug is dependent on the provision of intermediate services by the doctor and the chemist or druggist.

The importance of public institutions and non-profit making organizations in the provision of health care services in most economically developed countries was described earlier. Many health care services are not directly marketed to consumers but provided at zero or subsidized cost to the final consumer through direct public provision or funding of services. This distinction between marketed and non-marketed services is an important characteristic of many health care markets.

HEALTH CARE TECHNOLOGY AS A DYNAMIC PROCESS

The ways in which product and process innovations in technology have been analysed was described in Chapter 1. The main thrust of that research has been in tracing the growth of a specific technological innovation from inception to general acceptance within a manufacturing community. The framework commonly employed to describe this dynamic process of technological change has been to distinguish three phases: first the invention and generation of basic scientific knowledge, second the innovation by which these ideas are applied to the production of goods and services, and third the diffusion of these innovations amongst producers within an industry, across industries and between countries.

Invention and innovation

Some analyses of invention and innovation in manufacturing have incorporated data on health care technology, especially where innovations in drugs are concerned. Table 2.1 incorporates this data but augmented to include many more innovations in products and services in line with the substantially broader conceptualization of health care technology which has been described above.

There are a number of points which should be made concerning the data in Table 2.1. The information on invention and innovation outlined below confirms that health care is like other areas of product and service production in that there may be a considerable time lag between the identification of fresh knowledge and inventions and their application to health care production. Rutstein (1967) has argued that the history of health care highlights this type of time lag between invention and innovation. The reasons for this may be found in the identification of

Table 2.1 Basic innovations in health care technology

Type of technology	Invention	Innovation
Diagnostic technologies		
Stethoscope	Laennec 1819.	General adoption in America and Britain in 1850s. Improvements in original wooden instrument from 1820s onwards.
Microscope	Available in the eighteenth century but insufficient magnification. Chevalier 1823 and Lister 1830 improved the magnification.	Adoption in medicine and medical research from 1840s onwards.
Electron Microscope	1931.	1937.
Ophthalmoscope	Understanding eye/light interaction 1810. Helmholtz 1850.	Berlin 1850. Widespread adoption by late 1880s.
Laryngoscope	Bazzini device exploring body cavities.	Czermal 1857 rapid adoption.
X-ray	Photography 1850s. Roestgen 1895.	Improvements including Eastman Kodak X-ray film 1929. Quickly used in medicine. Established as routine diagnostic procedure in 1930s.
Electrocardiograph		Einthoven 1903.
Electroencephalograph		Berger 1929 with financial support from Carl Zeiss.
Computer	Von Neumann 1940s.	Biomedical use 1950s and general diagnostic aid 1960s.
CAT Scanner		Hounsfield 1972.

Table 2.1 *continued*

Type of technology	Invention	Innovation
Treatment technologies		
Anaesthesia	Understanding lungs and inhalation of gases 1770s/80s. Davy properties of nitrous oxide 1800.	Morton 1846 use in dental operations. Improvements in agents used – method injection 1884 – recovery of anaesthetic agent 1924.
Antisepsis	Development of germ theory, such as Bretonneau 1821 diphtheria transmission. Sassi 1835 sterilization of needles for vaccination. Pasteur process of fermentation 1850s. 1853.	Lister 1867 dressing material. Developed in surgical setting over next twenty years.
Aspirin		Bayer Company, Germany 1899.
Insulin	Banting 1920. Earlier work of Von Metiring and Minkowski 1899.	Banting and Best tests with human patients in 1922 and production in Canada and America in 1923. Improvement protamine insulin by Hagedorn 1933–5.
Anti malaria drugs	1932.	1932.
Sulpha drugs	Domagk prontosil 1932. Earlier work of Erhlich 'magic bullet' 1917.	1935 Sulphanilomide Farben Company, Germany. Many improvement technologies – chloromycetin, aureomycin and terramycin.

Table 2.1 *continued*

Type of technology	Invention	Innovation
Penicillin	Fleming 1929.	Florey and Chain isolate penicillin 1940. Production begins in 1944. Improvement technologies such as tetracycline 1947–53. Synthetic penicillin such as penbritin 1957–61.
Streptomycin	1924 Gratia, Dath and Rosenthal.	1943 Waksman and students. Production by Merck Company deep vat fermentation technique 1944. Improvements by Feldman through addition of further drugs 1948.
Cortisone	1931.	1948.
Psychotropic drugs		1952 reserpine. 1955 chloromazine. Early 1960s librium and valium. 1965 permate-nardil.

Disease prevention and health maintenance technologies

Vaccination		Arm to arm inoculation 1790s. Injection from 1884. Cell culture to propagate tissue cultures 1949.
Smallpox		Jenner 1790s.
Diphtheria		Antitoxin derived from Pasteur's work 1891.
TB		BCOG vaccines early 1900s. Waksman isolation. Streptomycin 1944 – widely available 1948 onwards and further drugs introduced.

Table 2.1 *continued*

Type of technology	Invention	Innovation
Rubella	Identified 1870s.	Meger and Parkman tested live vaccines 1966 – commercial production 1967.
Water supply and waste disposal		Sanitary reform movement of 1840s. Clean water supplies from local authorities in Britain and state and local government in America becoming widespread by the end of the nineteenth century. Introduction of the water closet in domestic housing.
Fluoridation	1930s studies linked fluorine and mottled teeth.	1941 Bibby, Tufts Dental School application of sodium fluoride to adolescents' teeth. 1945 controlled experiments on fluoridation of water supplies.
Contraceptive pill	1938 isolation of progesterone, sex hormone.	1954 contraceptive pill. Commercial manufacture by Searle in 1960.
Prevention of Rhesus Haemolytic	Clarke and Shepperd work on blood groups and rhesus factor 1953–60. Gorman and Pollock in America parallel work.	Clinical trials 1960–4.

Health organization and delivery technologies

Management/institutional

Diagnostic laboratory	1824–26 Rurkyne and Liebig laboratories.	Clinical laboratories in 1880s and ward laboratories in 1890s widely established in hospitals.

Table 2.1 *continued*

Type of technology	Invention	Innovation
Specialization		Emergence of specialization from 1870s with development of specialist organizations and publications.
Modern hospital	Paris hospitals of 1840s – design and organization.	The establishment of the hospital as the dominant institution in the system of health care from 1890s.
Group-based general practice	Mayo brothers 1890s.	The development of group practices and health centres in community-based health care from 1920s.
Computerization		Computerization of records for policy planning and service administration from 1960s.

Marketing

BRITAIN

Hospitals		Funding building of local hospitals 1860s/70s. Introduction of pay beds 1890s. Universal access through 1946 National Health Service Act.
General practice		Access in the population extended through (a) Friendly Societies especially by 1870s; (b) 1911 National Insurance Act; (c) 1946 National Health Service Act.

Table 2.1 *continued*

Type of technology	Invention	Innovation
AMERICA		
Hospitals		Introduction of pay beds 1890s onwards. Blue Cross 1929. Employer/union agreements through third-party insurers from 1940s. Medicare/Medicaid 1965.
General practice		Blue Shield 1930s. Employer/union agreements through third-party insurers from 1940s. Medicare/Medicaid 1965.
	Health centres run by voluntary agencies and municipal health departments 1910–15.	Health maintenance organizations 1960s.

Sources: Abbott, 1976; Boyle *et. al.*, 1985; Cartwright, 1977; Clark *et. al.*, 1983; van Duijn, 1983; Henwood and Thomas, 1984; Hough, 1975; Jewkes *et al.*, 1969; Kleinknicht, 1983; Reiser, 1978; Starr, 1982; Tarr *et al.*, 1984; Uttley, 1984; Williams, 1982; Wohl, 1983; Youngson, 1979. (A more specific consideration of the influence of political technologies upon changes in health care organization and delivery will be given in Chapter 4.)

the factors which affect the adoption and diffusion of innovations in health care and these will be discussed shortly. There may however be wider economic influences at work associated with the kind of economic changes suggested by long-wave theorists and these will be considered in Chapter 5. It is worth noting however that general links between social service innovation and economic cycles have been asserted before, for example by Heclo (1974, pp. 10–11) analysing innovation in incomee maintenance programmes. The general history of innovation also shows how basic innovations are frequently followed by a range of improvement innovations which improve the initial innovation or encourage complementary services and products. Health care shows a similar pattern: for example, the production of penicillin was followed by many improvements such as tetracycline and subsequently by the development of synthetic penicillin. Similarly the stethoscope was quickly transformed from Laennec's wooden instrument into the instrument we all recognize today. The change in the stethoscope was just a small part of the wider transformation of diagnostic techniques and the relationship between doctor and patient as new innovations and improvement innovations were introduced.

The process of identifying and dating innovations and distinguishing between basic and improvement innovations is a contentious one. Just as there are disputes outside the health care field about which innovations truly represent basic or radical innovations rather than improvements in existing products or processes, and the exact dating of inventions and innovations, so there are disputes in health care too. These disputes occur even in those areas of health which would appear easiest to identify such as the discovery and production of new drugs. These difficulties are not unexpected given the conception of invention and innovation as a process of 'cumulative synthesis' as defined by Usher (1954) and explained in Chapter 1. Attempts to date and describe these stages do give a valuable insight into the development of new technologies, but it is important to recognize the implicit limitations of classifying technological change into the three separate stages. As long as invention, innovation and diffusion are not seen as discrete phases, and the feedback effects of changes within a product or process change and between products and processes are recognized, then an insight into the complex process of 'cumulative synthesis' can be achieved.

The linkages between technical and social innovations have already been outlined. It was noted that innovations across a wide range of goods and services might cluster together around a single radical or basic technological innovation or small group of such innovations. This type of clustering of technologies can be seen within health care services, such as in the development of the hospital as the centre for treatment of acute health care problems since the late nineteenth century. Clustering may also involve innovations in technologies across a wide range of activities; for example, changes in personal transportation and communication systems have had an

important impact upon the availability, location and organization of general practitioner-based care in the community.

Diffusion of health care technologies

Chapter 1 included a review of the literature on the diffusion of
technological innovations in manufacturing and service industries, including diffusion within industries, between industries
and between countries. The overall pattern of innovation and
diffusion in health care follows the usual 'S' curve, with the
initial introduction of the innovation being followed by a rapid
growth in the adoption of the innovation and subsequently
improvement innovations and finally decreasing growth as the
potential of new improvements diminishes. The exact shape of
each 'S' curve will reflect the particular circumstances of each
innovation.

The various influences upon adoption can be summarized
under five major headings:

1   Production factors associated with the availability of capital,
    labour and natural resources.
2   Predicted level of demand for the product or service and the
    structural requirements necessary to realize the innovation.
3   Assessment of the technical feasibility of the innovation
    itself and its advantage over existing technology and any
    other alternative innovations.
4   The complexity of the innovation and hence the learning
    problems for staff associated with its adoption.
5   The compatibility of the innovation to the set of values held
    within the adopting organization and wider cultural values
    held in the community as a whole.

Economists have emphasized two main elements in the above
list which they regard as being of prime concern when decisions
about adoption are made: first, the assessment of the impact of the
innovation on the profitability of the organization, and, second,
the size of the capital requirements to realize the innovation. There
is no doubt that capital availability and profitability are important
in health care too, especially in the production of drugs and
medical products. Liebenau (1987, p. 31) has emphasized the

critical influence of the availability of capital, from banks and finance corporations, to the growth of manufacturing drug companies and distribution networks in America at the end of the nineteenth century and the early part of the twentieth century. It is also important to remember that the structure of the health care market frequently involves voluntary and public agency provision of health services and that government plays a pivotal role in the financing and regulation of such services. These structural features of the health care market will have a major impact on how profitability and capital generation are perceived in health care.

Research on diffusion in health care has mostly been concerned with the period after the Second World War. It is claimed that the rates of diffusion in health care have been extremely rapid and that this has been one of the major contributing factors to the escalation of health care expenditure in many countries during recent decades. Explanations for rapid diffusion of innovations have emphasized, first, changes in the level of demand for health care, including the structure of the health care market, and, second, the particular characteristics of health care organizations and the values espoused by both providers and consumers of health.

Changes in the size, composition and location of national populations have been regarded as important factors in the development of the welfare state as a whole and in individual social services such as health care (Boserup, 1981; Mishra, 1977). Changes in the size and structure of national populations, and the access to income within such populations, are important in affecting the level of demand which may be induced by the introduction of an innovation. Trease (1964) and Smith (1979) have shown how population and income growth were important in the diffusion of patent medicines in Britain and America towards the end of the nineteenth century. Linked with these developments was the growth of a much enlarged retail sector of chemists and druggists.

The level of demand is influenced not just by the cost of the service but also by the method through which payment is arranged. Historically this has been important in health care, for example in the evolution of the modern hospital where the introduction of direct payment in the form of 'pay beds' greatly increased access and usage of hospitals by the middle class. There seems to be considerable agreement amongst American researchers (Banta, 1981; Fuchs, 1986; Russell, 1979) that rapid diffusion of innovations in American health care has been substantially influenced by organizational innovations in systems of payment. This has been evidenced through the impact of Blue Cross, Blue Shield and employer/employee agreements with third-party insurers from the 1930s onwards and subsequently in public payments through Medicare and Medicaid from the mid-1960s. These innovations in the systems of payment for health care have played a major role in creating an environment in which basic and improvement innovations have been adopted with apparent ease in the American health system. The payment system may partially insulate patients and health care workers from questions of resource cost and risk assessment which accompany decisions about the diffusion of innovations in other areas of activity.

Perhaps equally as important as the influence of the level of demand for health services upon the diffusion of innovations is the range of values espoused by both providers and users of health care services. These values affect the total organizational environment, including the attitudes to learning amongst workers which are likely to be an important factor in the diffusion of innovations. The attitudes of professional workers in health care are important to an understanding of the diffusion of technologies because of the power which these workers exercise, especially over resource use decisions in relation to individual cases. The linkage between the physical sciences and medical sciences in the training and professional ideologies of health workers has already been noted. Medical science involves research and development in order to promote our understanding of illness and health. This understanding can then be translated into actions which it is said will improve the health status of individuals and communities. Professional and semi-professional workers in health care have gone through a similar process to that described by Mulkay (1972, pp. 19–24) in relation to the physical sciences. They have been socialized to accept a medical science perspective through formal education and similarly to accept the authority of professional associations.

Professional recognition in the form of tenure, or security of employment and promotion within the profession, depend upon generating knowledge and exchanging that knowledge with others. This exchange will occur both within a community of specialists, and within the profession as a whole, and at both a national and an international level. Learning is valued both as a goal in itself and for its instrumental value in terms of status and promotion. This emphasis upon learning amongst health care workers will probably influence their assessment of the learning requirements associated with the adoption and diffusion of a technological innovation. Overall professional attitudes are likely to encourage the rapid adoption of improvement innovations although they may be resistant to radical innovations which represent a break with the conventional professional perceptions which prevail towards a particular problem and potential solutions.

Provider pressures towards rapid diffusion may be further strengthened through providers responding to the attitudes of health care consumers. The health professions are caught by the success of their presentation of themselves to the public. The claim that through scientific endeavour all problems are susceptible to solution, and that 'new' ideas and therapies are constantly becoming available, encourages an expectation amongst consumers that treatments are always possible and that interventions will reflect 'state of the art' technologies (Blume, 1981). Consumer and media attention tends to be focused upon diseases which are life threatening, especially among the young and working adult population. The experience or fear of such illnesses among health consumers, which Schroeder and Showstack (1979) have described as the 'catastrophic illness' orientation, means that consumers with acute and severe chronic illnesses may place immense pressures upon physicians to try any treatment which might become available. David Banta (1981) has termed this the 'desperation reaction' in which a physician may use any innovation in an attempt to help the patient, irrespective of the lack of evidence to indicate whether the intervention is likely to help the patient or not.

The attitudes of health care workers and consumers towards new technologies is reflected in the values and practices of health care organizations. Schroeder and Showstack (1979, p. 190) suggest that hospitals are confronted with having to invest in new technologies in order to attract and retain physicians. Russell (1979, p. 150) provides support for this view through her analysis of technological diffusion in hospital care which indicates that larger hospitals, especially those which are committed to teaching and research activities, are the most likely to adopt innovations. This pressure to adopt innovations reflects the status of teaching and research activities and the need to be seen to produce new knowledge and techniques. Performance in respect to innovation is necessary to maintain public support in general and the support of those who provide the funding for research activities in particular. Blume (1981, pp. 110–11) argues that the rapid rate of diffusion in health care can be seen as a partial attempt to justify the level of public and private spending on research and development. Governments are important suppliers of research funding in health care both through public and private institutions and therefore these pressures can feed back into public health policy decisions.

One of the major factors influencing diffusion has been identified as the assessment of the feasibility of a technological innovation, both in a technical and financial sense. Whilst government regulations exist in most countries to ensure that innovations do not harm consumers, this does not ensure the efficacy of an innovation. Critics of the rate of diffusion in health care are implying that innovations are not adequately evaluated for their positive impact on health relative to either existing technologies or alternative innovations. Financial assessment of the profitability of innovations will be affected not just by the demand considerations already explained, but also by the fact that there are often relatively few suppliers of specific health care products and services in the market. The financial assessment will also be complicated by the importance of provisions which we have defined as intermediate goods and services to those who ultimately supply the service to the public.

There is debate in the literature as to what effect government intervention might have on the diffusion of health care technologies. Teeling-Smith (1980b), writing about the diffusion of technologies in the pharmaceutical industry, argues that safety standards are too stringent and discourage diffusion. Similarly he believes that government controls over prices and the advertising of drugs slow down innovation and impinge upon profitability of pharmaceutical companies. Grabowski (1980) has presented evidence to indicate that drug regulations in America have inhibited the speed of diffusion of new drugs originating from outside America into the American market. This inhibition of innovation has occurred even in those cases where there is ready agreement that the drug concerned would have a major beneficial therapeutic effect.

A very different approach however has been taken by Bice (1981) who sees changes in public regulation of health care as representing important innovations in health care in their own right. In the conceptual framework for health care innovations adopted in this book government regulatory changes would be seen as representing innovations in the political technology of health care within the wider category of changes in the organization and delivery technologies of health care. Changes in regulations will affect health care investment decisions, including the balance between capital and labour as the factors of production, and the direction and speed of technological change within the whole health care system.

Effective means of communicating the content of new innovations within an industry or service are important to the rate at which an innovation is adopted and diffused throughout an industry. The history of communication mechanisms in the diffusion of health care technologies has been well documented. Shryock (1960, pp. 117–33) has described how new ideas about many facets of medical knowledge and health care being generated in Paris during the early part of the nineteenth century were transmitted to America through Americans visiting and studying in Paris and Europe. These personal contacts were augmented by articles in foreign medical journals and through the writings of Americans, who had become familiar with the ideas emanating from Paris, writing in journals in their own country. The transmission and interchange of ideas about sanitary reform between America, Britain and Continental Europe during the middle of the nineteenth century, involved a similar process and has been described by Tarr and his colleagues (1984). Leavitt (1986, pp. 122–40) has described the way in which American doctors went to Germany during the latter part of the century to learn the Freiberg techniques of birthing including the administration of scopolamine. She documents how these doctors transmitted the Freiberg techniques amongst their colleagues upon their return to America.

In Chapter 1 it was noted that Ray (1984) claims that the diffusion of innovations is likely to take much longer where the capital requirements of an innovation are relatively low. This might be taken to imply that labour-intensive rather than capital-intensive innovations will be much slower to diffuse. Health care innovations do not necessarily entail low capital requirements; however, they do frequently require high labour input and this could be viewed as an inhibiting factor in the diffusion process. How can this observation be reconciled with the position taken by many writers that diffusion in health care occurs at a relatively rapid rate? The answer would seem to lie in the importance placed upon the exchange of ideas and information within professional health care occupations. There is competition to generate knowledge and technologies, but the dissemination of that knowledge is an intrinsic part of the process given that communicating new ideas is a critical component in the achievement of status and advancement in the health professions. There are long-established channels of communication in the professions by way of study arrangements, visits, conferences and journals. Improvements in national and international communications systems through international postal services, telephone and, more recently, fax and electronic mail facilities, represent a substantial process of enhancement and speeding up of longstanding exchange processes. The focus upon a highly developed learning environment by health care workers and organizations may be sufficient to overcome any impact which a labour intensive activity might have on the rate of diffusion of innovations. The communication mechanisms between health care workers may be sufficient to overcome the problems found in other areas of production of goods and services where information sharing is more difficult because of lack of common socialization and competitive restrictions.

EXAMPLES OF CHANGE IN HEALTH CARE
TECHNOLOGY

This chapter is concerned with technological change as a dynamic process and has used the framework of invention, innovation and diffusion of change as a helpful means of analysing such changes. This framework is further illustrated and discussed below in relation to selected aspects in the development of health care in America and Britain since the middle of the nineteenth century, namely the hospital, general practice and the pharmaceutical industry.

The rise of the modern hospital

Hospitals prior to the 1870s have been described as being based upon a 'refuge' approach (Smith, 1979, pp. 257–9) for the poor, homeless, immigrants, insane and illegitimate (Starr, 1982, p. 146; Vogel, 1979). This refuge was only extended to those who were regarded as deserving of such help when assessed against appropriate moral criteria, and some groups were commonly excluded; in Britain, servants, apprentices, pregnant women and children, for example (Woodward, 1974, pp. 45–50). Paradoxically hospitals were also thought of as places to store those whose moral weaknesses and misfortunes might spread through other sections of society (Vogel, 1980, pp. 62–4). The remoteness of many hospitals and the physical barriers of high walls and fences illustrate that the barriers to discharge were as real as the barriers to entry. The financing of hospitals came from the philanthropy of the wealthy, predominantly as individuals, or to a lesser extent in their role in local government bodies such as parish councils, municipal authorities or charitable organizations. Influence over many aspects of running the hospital was given to benefactors in return for their subscriptions. Subscribers could nominate patients for admission, exercise voting power in the administration of the hospital and in some cases had the right to inspect the hospital at any time (Woodward, 1974, p. 18). Physicians were, in the main, unpaid for their work within the hospital, but the reputation which they established for this work was an important factor in building up the patronage of their services from the wealthy who were treated and cared for by the physician within their own homes.

The number of hospitals and hospital beds in Britain and America grew considerably around the middle of the nineteenth century. In Britain there were about 4,000 hospitals in 1800 and this had grown to 11,848 by 1861 with the average length of hospital stay being between 30 and 40 days (Woodward, 1974, p. 31). In America the Civil War was the catalyst for a substantial building programme with the Union creating around 130,000 beds by the end of the war (Starr 1982, p. 153).

Hospitals were transformed by the early part of the twentieth century as Starr explains: 'in a matter of decades, roughly between 1870–1910, hospitals moved . . . from refuges mainly for the homeless poor and the insane, they evolved into doctors' workshops for all types and classes of patients' (p. 146). How did this transformation come about? Theoretical changes in medical knowledge which were generated in European schools, especially in Paris, became focused upon seeing the hospital as the appropriate centre for medical research and practice (Shryock, 1960). Ackerknecht (Waddington, 1973) argued that the hospital was the only site in which the three central pillars of the emergent medical science, namely examination, autopsy and statistics, could be successfully located. The bodies of those dying in Parisian hospitals became the property of the hospital administration and available for dissection if relatives did not pay a burial fee within twenty-four hours of notification. This practice, prior to the 1840s, gave physicians the right to examine the body of any patient dying in their care. The information obtained through examination of the body in autopsy was extremely important in promoting an understanding of anatomy and disease. Using these kinds of opportunities researchers such as Cruvelhier in Paris and Rokitansky in Vienna laid down the basis upon which modern pathological science is based.

The examination of the living, as well as the dead, became part of medical practice and involved a transition from passive observation and discussion with the patient to active physical examination. The adoption of physical examination both encouraged, and was encouraged by, innovations in diagnostic tools such as the stethoscope. These developments in Europe during the first half of the nineteenth century were diffused into Britain and America through the involvement of physicians in visits, study and writing.

The emphasis in the European schools was towards pursuing an understanding of the human body and the course of disease, rather than seeking treatment interventions as such. This increase in understanding, however, affected the potential for surgical interventions but improvements in surgery were dependent upon the introduction of two other innovations, namely anaes-thesia and antisepsis.

The properties of gases such as oxygen and the process of respiration had been the subject of discoveries towards the end of the eighteenth century. In the 1790s 'pneumatic medicine' involving the inhalation of gases was popular. In 1800 Davy examined the properties of nitrous oxide and its effect when inhaled but the relevance of this work to medicine was not taken up at this time. Hickman, a country doctor in Brit-ain, experimented using inhalation on animals but again this work attracted little attention. The beginnings of anaesthesia in medicine are usually attributed to two Boston dentists, William Morton and Horace Wells, who experimented with nitrous oxide and ether. In 1846 Morton used anaesthesia to perform surgery on a patient. Concern about the safety of ether led to a search for a better anaesthetic agent. Chloroform had been discovered by Soubeiran in France and Guthrie in America in 1831, and Simpson used, and established the anaesthetic effects of, chloroform in 1847. As with other types of innovation anaesthesia was subject to improvement innovations both in the agent used and in the techniques for administering the agent. Anaesthesia was gradually adopted in hospitals during the second half of the nineteenth century.

The development of antisepsis derived from an increasing understanding about how diseases were transmitted. At the end of the eighteenth century Gordon observed that puerperal fever could be transmitted from one patient to another by doctors and midwives. In 1821 Bretonneau discovered that diphtheria was caused by a specific germ and conjectured that diseases may have specific causes. Latour's work on yeast was developed in the 1850s by Pasteur's examination of fermentation processes and the role of minute organisms. This work was formalized in the germ theory of disease in 1864. Pasteur's work was further expanded by Koch who developed techniques for isolating and growing bacteria in a culture medium.

Technologies reflecting these developments in the medical understanding of disease were apparent from the 1830s. Bassi established the importance of sterilizing the needle used for inoculations by placing the needle in a flame. Lister, beginning in 1867, began to develop various types of dressing materials and agents to kill septic germs in surgical operations. Antiseptic techniques and agents were gradually developed and improved over the next fifty years. The techniques of asepsis, such as steam sterilization of instruments, surgical gloves, face masks and caps, were being introduced into hospitals towards the turn of the century (Cartwright, 1977; Youngson, 1979).

The gradual introduction of anaesthesia and antisepsis contributed to changes in the scope and impact of surgical interventions in hospitals even during the early years of introduction in the 1860s and 1870s. Woodward (1974, p. 76) notes a substantial increase in the number of operations at Leeds General in Britain from 179 in 1860 to 616 in 1875. Vogel (1980, pp. 60–1) states that the first operation using antiseptic techniques was performed at Boston Hospital in 1879 and that this technique and later asepsis became gradually established in the hospital. The range of possible surgical interventions and their impact was substantially changed by these innovations. From 1864 to 1869 about two-thirds of patients with compound fractures at Boston Hospital had a limb amputated and of these almost half died. But between 1889 and 1894 there were only eighty-two cases where amputations were performed and of these only fourteen died.

The advances in medical science which were generated in Europe during the nineteenth century changed the understanding of disease and led to advances in diagnostic techniques available for use within the hospital. The emergence of anaesthesia and antisepsis created opportunities for extending the range of possible surgical interventions and greatly increased the likely success of such interventions. The possibility of successful intervention was also extended by the innovation of an antitoxin for diphtheria in 1891.

The changes which established the hospital as the central institution of health care during the latter part of the nineteenth century were not confined to advances in medical knowledge and diagnostic and treatment technologies alone. Writers such as Abel–Smith (1964, p. 16), Woodward (1984, pp. 71–4) and Starr (1982, p. 146) have established that wider social changes such as population growth, urbanization and industrialization had a substantial influence upon the development of the modern hospital. Increases in the size and age structure of the population and in the concentration of that population in urban areas, combined with increases in per capita income and the effect of this on nutrition, were all factors affecting the growth in the numbers and size of hospitals (Woodward, 1984, pp. 70–5). Urbanization removed people from their informal networks of support, including access to the health care knowledge and skills which were held within family and local community structures, to which they had traditionally turned. Growing numbers of young people found themselves in boarding accommodation in burgeoning cities. Increases in longevity and decreases in family size were occurring alongside growing pressure on living space within an urban environment. These are some of the factors which placed pressure upon hospitals, especially at the turn of the century, to provide 'hotel' functions for many sections of the population (Vogel, 1979, pp. 110–16). Industrialization also influenced public attitudes towards health care in that there was general acceptance that it was necessary to look to specific occupations for specialist knowledge and competence in health production, just as had taken place in industrial production (Starr, 1982, p. 148).

Until the latter part of the nineteenth century hospitals had been perceived as institutions which were to be rightly feared by all sections of society. Smith says: 'The hospitals had a justified reputation as death-traps, the patients were cut off from their families and friends . . . the patients were peremptorily managed by underpaid, frightened and callous nurses' (1979, p. 246). Hospitals were frequently overcrowded with poor, dirty living conditions and inadequate food, and diseases were often spread from one patient to another in these circumstances. How serious these problems were in the sense of affecting survival rates within the hospital is disputed; for example, Woodward

(1974, pp. 121–6) has argued that the death rate in British hospitals might actually have been quite low.

The acceleration in the building of new hospitals and rebuilding of old ones began in the 1860s and accelerated in both Britain and America from the 1880s. This construction programme gave the opportunity to incorporate new ideas from medical science, including those concerning disease prevention and health maintenance technologies generated by the sanitary reform movement, in the physical design of the hospitals. New hospitals had hot and cold piped water supplies and the quality of that water was being vastly improved during the second half of the century in response to local government construction of new water supply systems. Open fires were replaced by alternative heating systems such as steam heating. Floors were no longer porous and the preparation of food was separated from patient care and especially from those with contagious diseases. Nickel-plated and enamelled instruments were introduced in the 1870s and subsequently steam sterilization techniques were gradually adopted.

The report on the administration of Paris hospitals in 1865 influenced the physical arrangement of patients within the hospital. From the 1880s hospitals were designed on the ward system in which patients were separated into groups based upon their condition. The idea of building special 'pavilions' for those with communicable diseases was also introduced (Rosen, 1963). The establishment of pavilion hospitals was a factor in the 'take off' of hospital growth in Britain (Pickstone, 1985, pp. 100–2), even though these ideas predated their scientific justifications in terms of germ theory and antiseptic techniques.

The rise of the hospital at the end of the nineteenth century as the central institution of health care services has been substantially influenced by innovations in scientific medicine. These innovations have, however, both influenced and been influenced by innovations in the way hospital services have been organized and delivered.

Changes in management and marketing of hospital services have been important in this respect. Prior to the 1860s funding and control over hospitals rested with the wealthy who provided voluntary subscriptions. In return for their subscriptions they received the right to nominate patients for entry into the hospital and also formed lay committees which exercised management control over the running of the hospital. Developments in the scope of work performed and in the organization of workers within hospitals led to changes in the management of hospitals.

Until the second half of the nineteenth century nurses had been recruited from those middle-aged women who had no family responsibilities and they were treated as servants or housekeepers. They were frequently regarded as being the 'worst sort of woman' (Woodward, 1974, pp. 30–5) and severe restrictions were placed upon their personal behaviour. Nursing care as such was often carried out by patients looking after each other. New ideas about the importance of physical care for the sick were closely related to the growth in medical knowledge which was being generated in Europe and concern as to how this knowledge could be realized in the hospital (Abel-Smith, 1964, pp. 50–64; Pickstone, 1985, p. 101). Florence Nightingale's ideas about nursing and nursing practice saw the beginnings of modern nursing in Britain with the first Nightingale training school at St Thomas's in 1860. Although the impact of training on the total structure of nursing was gradual, trained nurses exercised increasing influence as they rose to positions of hospital matrons in the late Victorian period. The involvement of religious orders of nuns in nursing within hospitals at this time also influenced the quality and quantity of nursing care. Similarly, in America, the first training school for nurses was established in 1873. The number of schools increased, usually centred in the hospital, and by the early 1920s about a quarter of American hospitals had a nursing school (Reverby, 1979). The emergence of nursing as a discrete occupation and of nursing training was important in improving the standard of physical care in hospitals from the 1860s. It was part of a change in focus within the hospitals towards 'reparation and care' (Smith, 1979, p. 258) which occurred prior to a further shift towards a scientific and clinical orientation from the 1880s.

Physicians practised in hospitals predominantly on an unpaid basis whilst seeking to establish their reputation and boost their practice outside the hospital through the patronage of wealthy patients who could afford to use the doctor's services within their own homes. Three major factors led to physicians seeking to stimulate hospital growth and exercise some degree of influence over the management of hospitals. Firstly, professional development, in the sense of improvements in the availability and quality of education and the formation of professional associations, led to demands being made upon hospitals to play an increasingly important role in the teaching process. The growth of medical education and the development of the modern hospital have been closely linked in the literature on health care services. Secondly, the increasing emphasis upon the scientific basis of medicine meant that there was a growing demand for opportunities for medical research. The hospital had become established in professional opinion within Europe as the most appropriate physical base for the development and practice of research in scientific medicine. Thirdly, the evolution of scientific medicine stimulated the development of specialization within medicine and physicians actively sought to pursue particular fields of research and practice. Changes in the way in which hospitals were organized, such as wards for specific conditions and laboratory facilities, assisted in the evolution of specialization.

Doctors were active in seeking the development of hospitals, and the management of hospitals gradually changed to reflect more closely the interests of doctors, and to a lesser extent of other workers like nurses. Initially a division in responsibility existed between on the one hand lay committees of subscribers and trustees who made decisions about hospital policy and on the other medical committees of doctors who were concerned with day to day decision making (Abel–Smith, 1964, pp. 33–8). The boundaries within this bipartite structure became less clear over time as doctors gained greater influence over decisions affecting their own working conditions and also over decisions on the handling of patients such as who would be admitted, the length of their stay and the discharge of patients. These changes reflected a recognition of the development of new knowledge and techniques in medicine which might create improvements in the outcome of health care interventions and which in turn conferred enhanced status on doctors.

In America the link between doctors and the hospital was further strengthened by the established manner of working which allowed community-based doctors to continue to treat their own patients when they entered hospital (Rosner, 1979; Starr, 1982, pp. 146–7). Rosner has estimated that in New York the practice of affiliating physicians to hospitals rose from 15.6 per cent in 1900 to 42.3 per cent in 1910; nationally, about two-thirds of doctors had staff appointments by 1928 and 83 per cent by 1933 (Starr, 1982, p. 165). This practice was not followed in Britain, nor in most parts of Europe, although the local general practitioner in Britain often had responsibility for the management of a local cottage hospital. As manager of this kind of small hospital a general practitioner was frequently in the position of being able to treat patients by virtue of this dual role.

In America, in particular, this period of increasing domination of management by doctors gave way to further developments which saw the emergence of an administrative class of specialist managers who did not have a medical background. The Association of Hospital Supervisors was formed in 1899, a university degree in hospital administration was initiated in the 1920s and the American College of Hospital Administrators formed in 1933 (Starr, 1982, p. 178). Hospitals were becoming more complex and the marketing of the hospital's services to the consumer, who increasingly made payments for the services received and to other organizations involved in the health care market, became more important (Perrow, 1979). Starr (1982, p. 168) has used Weber's notions of 'communal relations' and 'associative relations' to describe this transformation in health care in general and the organization of hospital care in particular. The hospital was transformed from being an institution based upon family, friendship and community ties founded on personal and group loyalties, to an institution which was based on economic exchanges which were derived from shared economic interests and ends.

The growing power of doctors in the management of the hospital was also apparent in the relationship between doctors and patients within the hospital. The transformation of the doctor-patient relationship, which was triggered by developments in diagnostic technologies, was described earlier in this chapter. Outside the hospital, doctors had relied heavily upon the wealthy for patronage of their services, and this somewhat dependent relationship circumscribed what interventions they could use. Experimenting with the use of diagnostic and treatment techniques, and indeed utilizing established techniques of examination, was problematical if they required physical 'access' to the body and therefore contravened social and sexual barriers. As Waddington (1973) pointed out in his analysis of the Paris Hospital, the fact that hospitals were the preserve of the poor and marginalized sections of society meant that doctors were able to exert domination over consumers in order to perform physical examinations of patients and demonstrate those examinations to students and other health workers. These practices would have been totally unacceptable to a doctor's patients outside the hospital. Equally, families of patients outside the hospital would have been unlikely to allow the bodies of their dead relatives to be used for dissection and the promotion of medical knowledge.

Changes in the manner in which hospitals were marketed to potential funders and consumers of hospital services are of considerable importance in accounting for developments in the hospital during the latter half of the nineteenth century and beginning of the twentieth century. The increase in hospital building in Britain during the 1860s has been attributed, in part, to the generation of increased donation income (Abel-Smith, 1964, p. 16). There were many innovations in fundraising techniques including social events like musical festivals and dinners. Hospital Saturday Funds began in the 1850s in Britain, encouraging working people to provide weekly subscriptions to the hospital, and shortly afterwards Hospital Sunday Funds were initiated which sought donations to local hospitals from church collections. These are all examples of the kind of innovative marketing techniques which played a part in increasing donation income (Woodward, 1974, pp. 19–21).

Towards the end of the century the marketing of hospital services changed dramatically. The economic depression of the late 1870s and 1880s placed a considerable strain upon hospital funding and in addition public perceptions of hospitals were being transformed in the light of advances in diagnostic and treatment technologies. As Abel-Smith puts it: 'More hospital accommodation was needed because improvements in both medicine and nursing were making it more advantageous for the sick to be admitted' (1964, p. 152). The demand for hospital services was increasing at a time when hospital costs were rising (Rosner, 1979, p. 118) and hospital income was under pressure. Hospitals had not generally charged patients for their services as their patients were predominantly poor and unable to pay. From the 1880s onwards hospitals in both Britain and America introduced further marketing innovations which saw new packages of services introduced aimed at encouraging the use of hospitals by a much wider section of the community and these packages frequently entailed some form of patient charges (Abel-Smith, 1964, p. 150; Smith, 1979, p. 284). Groups such as trade unions and friendly societies took collective action in response to changing attitudes to hospitals and sought to establish mechanisms which would enable their members to have access to hospitals' facilities. The growing importance of payments can be illustrated by data from New York where, in the decade from 1911 to 1921, the percentage of patients who were private patients, or made payments of some kind, doubled, and by 1922 patient payments accounted for 65.2 per cent of the income of general hospitals (Starr, 1982, pp. 160–4).

Hospitals, in their role as centres for medical research, began to use that research work to seek funding from both companies and government whilst holding out the promise of further advances in treatments and growth in usage of the hospital. Pickstone (1985) has described how scientific 'breakthroughs', such as the discovery of X-rays and their use in diagnosis, were used by hospitals to solicit financial support. The emphasis on commercial marketing of hospital services was particularly strong in America. Reverby (1979) has described American hospitals as centres of business and scientific advancement by the beginning of the 1920s. The 'success' of the hospital can be seen in the dramatic growth in both the numbers and size of hospitals over a fifty-year period. In 1873 in America there were 178 hospitals, but by 1910 there were 4,000 hospitals and their size had increased. In 1923 there were 6,830 hospitals and one-third of these had nursing schools attached to them.

These links between increasing hospital usage and innovations in product and marketing technologies in health care is still evident in contemporary debate. In America the number of hospital beds and personnel have grown by over 50 per cent since 1960 (Altman and Wallack, 1979). This sustained growth in the size of hospitals has been attributed to two main influences; first, the introduction of new technologies such as intensive care units, and second, the sustained growth in the coverage and extensiveness of third-party insurance payments (Schroeder and Showstack, 1979; Stoman, 1976).

Aspects of general practice medicine

Prior to the late nineteenth century, practising medicine within the community was not a particularly lucrative occupation, except for a small elite group, nor were doctors held in particularly high social standing. Many doctors in fact practised several occupations concurrently in the seventeenth and eighteenth centuries in order to make a living. In both America and Britain general practice grew out of the role of apothecaries whose dominant activity was dispensing and selling drugs rather than giving advice on health problems. The numerous radical innovations in scientific medicine, which were important in transforming the hospital, were neither available directly to general practitioners nor through the testing facilities provided by hospital laboratories until well into the twentieth century. Many of the diagnostic techniques of auscultation, measurement of body temperature and blood pressure only gradually came into use in community medicine. The treatment technologies of modern drugs, which have figured so prominently in general practice in the second half of the twentieth century, have become available from the mid-1930s onwards. Organizational changes did occur around the middle of the nineteenth century. Doctors took collective action through the formation of professional bodies with the British Medical Association being formed in 1836 and the American Medical Association in 1846. These bodies, however, did not begin to exercise a major influence upon health care services until the latter half of the century.

Just as hospital services for much of the nineteenth century were confined to the poor so doctors practising in the community predominantly served those who could afford to pay for their services which were delivered to patients in their own homes. The operation of 'sick' clubs, friendly societies and action by a few employers to provide health care at the workplace for employees afforded a limited expansion in access.

Some doctors extended access to selected patients by providing services at no cost or subsidizing services to the poor by increasing the level of fees charged to wealthy patients. Another important influence upon increasing access to health care was the effect of high rates of economic growth towards the end of the nineteenth century. Growth was reflected in increased levels of personal incomes which improved the ability of people to afford to consume health care.

In Chapter 1 the idea that important new technologies may occur in 'bundles' or 'clusters' was acknowledged: that once the infrastructure required for such innovations is in place then there may occur a series of other innovations across quite a wide range of activities. Communication costs, especially the cost of transport, have been identified as a major barrier to the extension of access to general practitioner services in the latter half of the nineteenth century. Starr (1982, pp. 67–8) estimates that the charge by a doctor for travelling five to ten miles to visit a patient would cost four or five times the fee for the medical service entailed in the visit. A cluster of communications innovations and infrastructure investments dramatically changed communication networks from about 1880 to 1920. Personal communication was transformed by the creation of railroad transportation between cities and from rural areas to urban areas. The invention of the automobile engine in 1885 and the development of assembly line production from 1913 led to the development of much improved road structures and dramatic changes in personal transportation. The invention of the telephone in 1881, switchboards in 1892 and the telegraph in 1900 allowed direct and speedy interpersonal communication. These innovations, alongside the increasing concentration of population in urban areas, meant that the speed and ease of communication between potential patients and doctors was much enhanced. The cost of the communication component in the community doctor's service was also dramatically decreased. This cluster of communications innovations initially changed the ability of doctors to provide services to their patients in their own homes and at a cost which more people were able to afford. One of the effects of these changes was that doctors became much less reliant upon a small group of wealthy patients. In the longer term improvement innovations in both the products – cars and buses – and the processes by which they were produced led to widespread dissemination of cheap public and personal transport. Access to personal and public transport gradually allowed doctors to require patients to visit their surgeries rather than the doctor having to visit the patient.

Some of the innovations in organization and delivery of health care in hospitals have been mirrored in general practice. The increase in the size of hospitals and the continual development of specialization within the hospital have had parallels in general practice. The invitation of the Mayo brothers to other local general practitioners to join with them in serving their neighbourhoods in New York saw the initiation of private group practice at the end of the nineteenth century. By 1914, when they opened a new building to house the clinic, there were seventeen doctors and eleven clinical assistants involved in the practice. Guthrie, who had worked at the Mayo clinic, opened his own clinic in Sayre, Pennsylvania, in 1910. By 1932 there were over 300 group practices in America, usually with five or six doctors and geographically concentrated in the middle and far west (Starr, 1982, pp. 210–12). The movement towards forming larger units within general practice allowed doctors to seek some of the perceived advantages of their hospital counterparts. These included a move toward specialization and establishing the community practice as a centre for medical education. The group practice also came to be viewed as the most appropriate location for the work of other health workers such as nurses, midwives, social workers and physiotherapists.

In discussing the hospital it was noted that American and British general practitioners were placed in quite different positions in respect to their relationship with the hospital. General practitioners in America have been able to be formally linked with a hospital and through this link to treat their own patients when hospitalization is necessary. In Britain the division between general practice and hospital doctors is much more sharply drawn. This division dates back to the distinction between the work of physicians and surgeons on the one hand and that of apothecaries, from which general practice evolved, on the other. The Dawson Report (Consultative Council on Medical and Allied Services of the Ministry of Health, 1920) was important in reinforcing this distinction in that it saw a comprehensive health service as incorporating two major elements, a specialist service based in the hospitaal and a general service available to patients in their homes. The general practitioner represented the link between 'home'- and 'hospital'-based services. This linkage however did not entail direct involvement in the hospital service but rather the assessment of whether the specialist hospital service was required and the likely area of specialty needed. General practitioners were physically excluded from direct service within the hospital and have been confined to a limited treatment role. They act as the portal through which consumers must pass to gain access to the diagnostic and treatment knowledge of specialist staff.

The impact of these differing organizational technologies is well illustrated in the development of community-based medicine. In America the first specialty practice board was established in 1916. During the next fifty years the number of boards increased to twenty and the number of specialties to thirty. The impact on general practice has been dramatic. In 1931 80 per cent of physicians were in general practice but by 1966 75 per cent of physicians were in specialty practice of some kind (Sidel, 1971, pp. 165–7).

Earlier in this chapter the idea that scientific medicine might not only be able to 'read' the individual body but also the 'social body' was described. General practice is central to the extension of medicine outside the walls of the hospital and directly into the community to locate those most vulnerable to ill health. Many organizational innovations in community medicine in the twentieth century have confronted the problem of how to achieve effective links with those most vulnerable to health problems within the community. One of these innovations has been the health centre movement which was popular in many countries including America, Britain, Russia, Yugoslavia and Chile from the early part of this century until the 1930s. A number of centres were formed in America in the 1910–15 period. They were usually financed by local taxes or by philanthropy or a combination of the two and run by voluntary agencies or municipal health departments. They were focused particularly on the poor and aimed to make health care more accessible and to involve the local community in the running of the service (Stroeckle and Candib, 1974). In Britain the famous Peckham Health Centre experiment began in 1926 and offered regular monitoring of individual health. By the time of the second stage of the experiment in 1935 the emphasis had changed to how healthy living might be achieved and promoted and seeking a family rather than an individual focus for the service. The underlying ideas included the belief that everyone might potentially become ill, or at least not maintain good health, unless subject to regular monitoring and advice. It was also felt that the health care needs of the individual could only be understood in the context of the living group in which he or she was a member. These ideas and their realization are part of what Armstrong (1983, pp. 57–8) has referred to as the 'technologies of surveillance'.

Although health centres in America declined from the 1930s, and in Britain never developed in the 1920s and 1930s as had been envisaged in the Dawson Report, many of the ideas behind the health centre movement have subsequently reappeared with various modifications in the organization of general practice during the 1960s and 1970s. In Britain the idea of the 'health care team' incorporating many health care workers was supported in the Gillie Report (Central Health Services Council, Ministry of Health, 1963). These teams would involve bringing a wide range of services much nearer to the local communities in which the team operated. The growth of health centres in Britain has been a gradual process with only 100 centres being established between 1948 and 1968. Changing attitudes towards centres combined with changes in the system of funding led to an increase in the number of centres to 800 by 1975, although this still involved only about 20 per cent of all general practitioners (Levitt, 1977). In America similar ideas have been evident in the neighbourhood health centres which developed following the 1964 Presidential Commission on Heart Disease, Cancer and Stroke and in health maintenance organizations which were sanctioned through enabling legislation in 1971. These schemes have incorporated organizational innovations through local community participation in management and the monitoring of the health status of local populations.

Pharmaceutical industry

The public perception of the modern pharmaceutical industry is probably of an enterprise based upon high levels of research and development which is closely aligned to the general search for scientific and medical knowledge. The industry is seen as being based upon high levels of product innovation and a public expectation that new 'miracle' drugs will be discovered through research efforts within the industry. If the development of the industry since the beginning of the nineteenth century is examined it can be seen that it is not just product innovations which have been important. Technological innovations in the process of production and in management and marketing innovations have also been extremely influential.

The production of medicines in the first half of the nineteenth century was a relatively simple task, both with regard to the main drugs used by doctors and apothecaries at that time and the various 'miracle' potions and pills such as Morrison's Pills or Beecham's Powders in Britain. The raw materials necessary for manufacture were imported into Britain by companies such as the East India Company. These basic materials and the necessary manufacturing equipment were exported on to America for the production of drugs there. Wholesalers sold the raw materials which were few in number to chemists, druggists and doctors for preparation for use by consumers. During the second half of the century the wider social changes of growth in population size, urbanization and the increase in the level of per capita income not only had an impact upon access to health care in general but also to drugs. This was demonstrated by a dramatic increase in the sale of patent medicines. Smith (1979, p. 345) estimates the number of patent medicine sales in Britain in 1880 at well in excess of 17 million and there was a fourfold increase in the number of licensed vendors of medicines from 10,000 in 1865 to 40,000 in 1905 (Chapman, 1974). Liebenau (1987, pp. 10–25) has described the expansion in pharmaceutical manufacturing in America after the civil war. This expansion included increases in the number of medicines being produced, in the number of people employed in the industry and in the level of capital investment.

In both Britain and America major innovations were occurring in the organization of the industry. Many of the druggists and chemists moved into wholesaling of medicines and later some developed into major manufacturers of drugs. They adopted technologies that were being developed in other sectors of the economy for manufacturing and distribution. The manufacture of a wide range of acids, alkalis and salts was an essential element in the industry and some pharmaceutical firms at this time moved on to general chemical manufacturing. The pharmaceutical firms which emerged were initially owned by a particular family or group of families but by the beginning of the twentieth century these firms were passing into the control of management hierarchies with access to wider sources of capital funding and demonstrating increasing size and complexity. The importance of the knowledge being generated by scientific medicine through the work of researchers such as Pasteur and Koch was being recognized in the industry. The diffusion of this knowledge within the pharmaceutical industry came through improved relations with the medical profession and in America the influence of doctors' direct contact with European medical schools as well as journals. Small pharmaceutical wholesalers in America began to employ both scientific and medically trained staff at around the turn of the century. Research laboratories were set up, although at this stage their main purpose was not the development of new products but the standardization and testing of existing medicines.

During the first twenty or thirty years of this century a number of important process innovations, which had first become available from the middle of the nineteenth century, were utilized in the pharmaceutical industry. These included the use of the power loom in the production of surgical dressings and the utilization of steam sterilization techniques. American innovations, such as the compressed pill in 1843, the 'tablet' in 1878 and the rotary tablet machine in 1903 were instrumental in the realization of mass production techniques and transforming consumption from the point of view of the recipient of medication. The marketing of drugs was also affected by changes in the organization of drug retailing as larger organizations of chain drugstores and chemists were formed. These chain retailers covered more extensive geographical areas and had greater buying power in their negotiations with wholesalers and manufacturers.

The mid-1930s and 1940s represent the period of very rapid product innovations associated with the discovery of the sulpha-based drugs and penicillin-based antibiotics. In Britain the output of the pharmaceutical industry between 1935 and 1948 increased by over 400 per cent (Reekie, 1975, pp. 7–8). The realization of such an output growth depended not just upon the identification and isolation of each of the new drugs, but also on the availability of suitable production technologies. Reekie (1975) specifically cites the use of fermentation techniques, expertise in the production of dyestuffs and general chemical-processing technologies as being central to the ability to expand pharmaceutical output in the 1940s and 1950s. The therapeutic drug revolution is another example of the clustering of innovations across several types of activity which appears to be frequently required for the realization of a specific set of innovations.

3 Production, Consumption and Health Care Technology

In the previous chapter technological change in health care was portrayed as a dynamic process in which the generation of scientific knowledge and invention was applied to health. Invention generates innovations in both the content of health services and in the manner in which they are made available. These innovations become diffused within health care systems and various improvements are made to innovations so that their potential benefits can be fully realized. Having examined technological change as a dynamic process it is now possible to explore how innovations affect the manner in which health care is produced and consumed.

LOCATION AND CONTROL

As has already been described, for most of the population in Britain and America access to professional medicine was not readily available until the twentieth century. Health care was largely produced within the confines of the domestic economy with women being expected to play the central role in providing care for household members. Support for domestic production came through a variety of informal networks within local communities. Advice and direct help might be provided through these networks, especially from older women within the community who had acquired a reputation in the locality for their skills in dealing with health problems. Another source of health care advice to the household came from printed medical guides, such as William Buchan's *Domestic Medicine*, which were very popular in the late eighteenth and nineteenth centuries. These manuals presented an overall view of illness in which the primary reason for ill health was to be found in the behaviour of the sick person. By avoiding sinful and immoral behaviour people could exert some degree of control over their own health. Illness was not generally regarded as requiring professional intervention.

Some alternative health care practitioners, such as Samuel Thompson in New England, proclaimed the importance of conveying knowledge about health to everyone rather than allowing that knowledge to be controlled by a few people (Starr, 1982, p. 53). Figures such as Thompson were part of what Starr refers to as 'popular medicine' and comprised a wide variety of healers and therapists. Patent medicines which claimed to relieve many illnesses, such as Morrison's Pills, Beecham's Powders and Lydia Pinkham's vegetable compound, became available from the late 1820s. As has already been noted the sale of patent medicines such as these grew rapidly towards the end of the century. This growth partially reflected the role which patent medicines played in the production of health within the household, given that the use of a doctor's services might be seen as neither desirable nor affordable.

Industrialization transformed the overall basis of the domestic economy by removing the location of production of goods, and to a lesser extent services, from the household to the factory. The increasing concentration of population in urban areas in order to meet the labour requirements of factory-based production also affected the capacity of the household to meet the health needs of its members. The effects were felt through their impact upon extended family and local community networks. These effects included changes in domestic living arrangements, with a substantial growth in the numbers of single people, especially young single people, living on their own in the city and increasing geographical mobility as people sought to retain employment.

The transfer of health production from the household to specialist institutions was a gradual process which took place throughout the second half of the nineteenth century and the beginning of the twentieth century. The reasons for this gradual change are complex and varied but change in the technological base of health care production was a necessary element in making such a transition possible. The basic innovations in diagnostic and treatment technologies which characterized the development of scientific medicine in the nineteenth century required social innovations in the management, marketing and social and political organization of health care before they could be fully realized. For many sections of the population health care remained within the domestic economy throughout much of the nineteenth century.

During the nineteenth century the attitudes of working-class and middle-class households towards formal medical care from doctors in both hospital- and community-based practice were characterized by distrust. The move towards acceptance of changing explanations concerning the nature of illness and disease, which were being generated by scientific medicine, and a belief in the potential capacity of those with formal medical training to influence the course of an illness, took time to be disseminated and to modify attitudes within the population. Even when the value of formal medicine became more widely accepted the ability of many sections of the population to afford medical care awaited increases in per capita incomes. Access also depended upon innovations in communications systems and organizational innovations in health care services which did not become established until well into the twentieth century.

In the nineteenth century the wealthy had been able to purchase the services of a physician. The service was based in the domestic economy in the sense that physicians treated patients in their own homes. Control over production was not located entirely in the hands of the doctor, however. As many writers (such as Waddington, 1973; Woodward, 1984) have observed, doctors relied upon the patronage of wealthy patients. The combination of service location and service purchase meant that these patients were in a position to exert some degree of control over the way the service was made available to them and play a part in determining what was an acceptable treatment.

One of the effects of industrialization was to change the position of women in wealthy and upper-class households. Towards the middle of the nineteenth century they gained a measure of influence over how the domestic household was run and in the education and personal health of family members. Just as women have been identified as the central figures in domestic health production prior to industrialization, so they were instrumental in transferring many of these functions to formal health care systems during the next hundred years. They were active in the creation of reform movements which sought to improve a wide variety of services for themselves and their children (Verbrugge, 1979).

This transformation is well illustrated by an examination of the way in which childbearing practices have changed since the beginning of the nineteenth century. Leavitt (1986) has described childbearing in America during the eighteenth and nineteenth centuries as a service produced within the informal domestic economy and clearly controlled by women. Pregnant women turned to female relatives, experienced women in the local community and predominantly female midwives to deal with the birthing process in the mother's own home. Male midwives were known from the middle of the seventeenth century. In Britain they tended to charge more for their services and there was a status element in their attendance, which became apparent during the nineteenth century as prominent figures such as Queen Victoria used the services of a male midwife.

There is some indication that a division of work occurred between male and female midwives in both America and Britain. Male midwives were often brought in to help where there were difficulties being experienced in the birth and tools such as forceps, hooks, loops and knives were required (Osherson and AmaraSingham, 1981, pp. 232–7; Towler and Bramall, 1986, p. 113). These types of mechanical interventions were only rarely used. Smith (1979, chapter 1) has estimated that about 8–10 per cent of births in the 1860s in Britain might have involved these kinds of interventions. The use of tools such as forceps was later to become a common feature of birthing in the middle of the twentieth century. Osherson and AmaraSingham (1981, pp. 232–4) describe this division of labour in health care, linking active mechanical interventions with male work and passive interventions with female work, as part of a wider social change through which a perception of male control over machines became established. Despite these developments in mechanical intervention, male birth attendants and doctors were only used by the wealthy who could afford their services. Their role was still limited to that of *accoucheur* in which they did not displace the female midwife. They were also under the direction of the attendant women, who were drawn from within the local community and family structure, and who retained control at this stage over the birthing process.

The transfer of childbirthing from the home to the hospital, and from the control of women to the control of the medical profession, was influenced by the same technological innovations which were instrumental in the emergence of the modern hospital. Leavitt (1986) has documented the pressure which women's reform movements placed upon doctors to apply the innovation of anaesthesia, and its various improvement innovations, to childbirth during the nineteenth century. The possibility of reducing both the fear of pain and the actual experience of pain during labour meant that women both individually and collectively sought to have access to anaesthesia. Interest in the German Freiburg technique, including the use of scopolamine rather than chloroform or ether, attracted many American doctors to go to Germany to learn these techniques. The use of what became known as the 'twilight sleep' technique meant that women did not experience pain during childbirth but often had no mental recollection of their labour. In both America and Britain there was resistance to the adoption of anaesthesia as a regular feature of childbirthing and this affected the speed of diffusion of the innovation. Women activists accused doctors of withholding access to substances which would help women and claimed that the decision on using an anaesthetic agent should be the mother's and not the doctor's.

Opposition to the use of anaesthesia in childbirthing came from doctors. On the basis of available evidence they questioned the safety of the available anaesthetic agents, the techniques of administration and the adoption of anaesthesia as a universal method. The deaths of several women under anaesthesia, including a prominent campaigner in the twilight sleep movement, also raised public concern about safety. Smith (1979) describes the existence of opposition on moral grounds which focused on the morality of removing pain during labour and fears of possible sexual misconduct which might occur whilst women were anaesthetized. These fears are examples of more general obstacles to scientific medicine where innovations in diagnostic and treatment techhniques meant that doctors had to transgress existing social and sexual taboos surrounding touching. Despite opposition, the use of anaesthesia became well established in childbirth practice. In 1900 about 50 per cent of births in America involved both anaesthesia and a physician attending at the birth.

The majority of births remained located in the home until well into the twentieth century. In America about half of all births took place in hospital by the 1920s (Osherson and AmaraSingham, 1981, p. 235) but in Britain the adoption of hospitalization was slower, with 85 per cent of births still taking place in the home in 1927 (Towler and Bramall, 1986, p. 210). Changes in public attitudes towards the hospital through the recognition of the potential of various innovations in diagnostic and treatment technologies took time to diffuse among the population. Antisepsis techniques did not become well established in the hospital until the beginning of the twentieth century and fear of death and illness stemming from infection within the hospital remained strong. Ironically the increasing levels of intervention in home births, through anaesthesia and mechanical interventions such as forceps, increased the risk of infection during home births and led to arguments in favour of hospital births based on providing a safer environment. Surgical intervention in childbirth through Caesarean section was dependent upon anaesthetic and antisepsis techniques and was not widely used until the twentieth century. This technique did offer another option for intervention and one which was more aligned with the types of interventions that were seen as appropriately located in the hospital. Improvements in the standard of nursing care in hospitals which began in the 1860s and 1870s continued into the twentieth century. There were other improvements in the quality of the environment in the hospital, for example in the level of comfort afforded in the many new hospital buildings and the quality of services such as meals within hospital.

Leavitt (1986) argues that it was the twin influences of a growing belief in the efficacy of scientific medicine and specialist knowledge and increasing concern about the apparent deficiencies in familial and community networks in providing care, or at least in matching the perceived improved standards of care within the hospital, which led to the widespread transfer of childbirth from the home to the hospital. Middle-class women were in the forefront of those advocating hospital births during the 1920s and 1930s because the hospital was seen as offering the 'safest application of the newest technological and scientific methods of birth' (Leavitt, 1986, p. 171). By 1950 almost 90 per cent of births in America took place in hospital and by the 1960s births outside hospital were quite rare. Hospital births took off in Britain in the wake of the creation of the National Health Service in 1948 following a gradual increase from the beginning of the century.

The mechanization of childbirth became more extensive and sophisticated as the hospital was established as the dominant site for births to take place. The use of forceps in delivery became an established feature of birthing practice during the 1930s and 1940s. There were advances in pain relief both in terms of the agents available and the techniques for administering them. Monitoring of mothers during pre-natal care and during labour has become increasingly extensive, allowing the detection of possible birth abnormalities and the identification of the gender of the baby prior to birth. Techniques to control the onset and speed of labour became available and established as a common feature of childbirthing so that 'production' could be matched to the capacity of the hospital at any point in time. Childbirth has developed into a highly mechanized process which is controlled by professional and technical staff within the hospital. Just as women in the nineteenth and early twentieth centuries played an important role in influencing changes in childbirth practice so childbirth has remained an important focus for political action by women since the 1950s. The treatment of birth as a technical event which is controlled by doctors, technicians and machines is at the centre of dispute in contemporary debate. Alternative technologies have been advocated by many women's groups including a return to home-based deliveries in which women would again collectively exert control over production.

Childbirth practices represent a clear illustration of how health care services have been transferred from the realm of the domestic household economy, and in this case the control of women, to institutions within the formal health care system in which services are controlled by workers from professional and managerial occupations. There are many influences that have affected this transformation but an understanding of the change has to take into account the impact of technological innovations, not just in scientific medicine, but also in the ways in which these services have been organized and delivered.

It is interesting to note in passing that the contrast between production within the household economy and within the industrial factory or service institution may not have been as marked as it might first appear. Joyce (1980, chapter 2) has described how families were employed in various occupations within the factory or mill and how both familial and local community relations were often replicated within the factory. In the previous chapter hospitals in the nineteenth century were described as being based on 'communal relations'. These networks featured mutual caring between patients, support from family members, community involvement in financing and philanthropic giving from groups of wealthy local people. It might be thought that the transformation of the hospital into the site of production of health care under the control of professional and managerial elites would have removed the influence of communal relations. In many ways familial influence was eliminated. This is perhaps most clearly demonstrated by the strict control exerted over which family members could visit a patient in hospital, when they could visit and the careful monitoring of what happened during visits. Unlike some factories which brought family structures directly into the workplace along with the members of the family, hospitals created substitute family structures. The hospital superintendent represented the 'father' figure and the matron the 'mother' and both workers and patients were treated as part of a strictly hierarchical family (Reverby, 1979). Despite the developing scientific sophistication of medicine within the hospital, and the growth of professionalization and managerial skills needed in a complex institution, the notion of the hospital as a 'home' in which the 'family' of workers and patients lived was still a powerful feature of hospital organization until the 1940s and 1950s. The hospital has not been peculiar within social service institutions in using this replication of family structures in its organization. The use of this organizational strategy may have assisted the diffusion of more formal systems of service production in health and other social services through diminishing the effect of any clash in cultural values involved in transferring personal services from the family to the 'factory'.

TECHNOLOGICAL CHANGE AND THE FACTORS OF PRODUCTION

Capital

The decision to develop an invention and adopt any consequent innovation is influenced by an assessment of the rate of financial return on an investment and the availability of capital. In what ways has capital commitment in health care influenced the pattern of technological change in health services?

The transformation of hospital and general practitioner services in the nineteenth and early twentieth centuries was described in the previous chapter. Health care was removed from the realm of the household, in which both household members and doctors and other health workers had had a part to play, and into the realm of institutions such as hospitals and group general practice. The numbers of hospitals increased as did their size and complexity. This process of concentration in the organization of hospital services, in both public and private sectors, has continued until the present day. The hospital, as the centre of health care production, became the equivalent of the factory and displayed similar features. An increasingly complex pattern of specialization developed both between and within hospitals. Managerial and professional elites became established and began to exercise considerable influence over the functioning of the hospital. In time similar features became apparent in the organization of community health care through group practice, health centres and more recently the emergence of health maintenance organizations in America.

The health care system of the nineteenth century required relatively little capital investment beyond modest amounts of land, bricks and mortar for the building of hospitals. Innovations in scientific medicine dating from the middle of the nineteenth century onwards have generated an ongoing need for greater capital commitment. The size of the hospital thought necessary to provide a focal point for scientific medicine has become larger and the equipping of such a hospital more complex and capital-intensive. The growing capital requirements of the hospital have been a response to changes in treatment and diagnostic technologies and the related increased demand for hospital services.

A similar trend has been apparent in general practice as the service moved from a home based service to a distinct site in a local geographical community in which several doctors and other health workers frequently work. Specialization took place between doctors, and between doctors and other workers. Access to specialist support services outside the general practice, in order to analyse diagnostic tests, became established as a necessary feature of community practice.

The movement of health care in both hospital and community medicine to mirror product manufacturing in the factory is related to the changes in the position of the health care consumer which were described in Chapter 2. The consumer's role was gradually changed from one of active and equal participation in the service to passive receipt of a service controlled by health care workers. Consumers have come close to being mere 'inputs' in the service generation process.

In Chapter 1 various economic influences upon the adoption and diffusion of technological innovations in products and processing in manufacturing were described. The two factors which were identified as being of particular importance in any decision to adopt an innovation and proceed with development were the level of perceived risk and the likely rate of profitability. The factors influencing capital investment decisions in health care have historically been quite distinct, and certainly more complex than those operating in product manufacturing.

Philanthropic giving by the wealthy has been an important source of capital for the development of hospital-based health care in both America and Britain. Philanthropy cannot by any means be regarded as totally divorced from self-interest. Self-interest is manifest in expressions of concern about the impact of philanthropic giving upon the social and political status of benefactors and in attention to any indirect financial benefits which may come from giving. Philanthropy, however, is at least partially a reflection of concern for others as well as self-interest and is definitely not grounded on narrow assessments of profit levels and managing risk in capital commitment (Uttley, 1980). In a similar manner the donation of funds through local geographical communities has also been a critical source of capital in the founding of local hospitals and other community health care services. Community giving has been partially based on altruism as well as self-interest and has certainly not relied solely on 'enforced' payments imposed through national and/or local taxation systems.

Non-profit-making organizations and church-based agencies have provided in the past, and continue to provide in the present, important health care services within most health care systems. Their investment decisions may reflect a wish to ensure that service costs are recovered and that there are sufficient funds for reinvestment or to devote to other activities. In either case the decisions on capital investment have wider parameters than just the rate of return or associated risk. Such organizations have also been characterized as more likely to innovate than either public or private sector providers. An acceptance of this image of being leaders rather than laggards in technological innovation in social services may be an important element in capital commitment decisions which promote the adoption and diffusion of innovations by this type of organization. The decision is partly a reflection of the culture of the organization which is constructed through the interaction of both internal and external factors.

Decisions about capital investment are likely to be further complicated by the role of the public sector complex in health. The substantial contribution which governments make to research and development costs in health care, including pharmaceutical, has already been noted. Governments commonly play the role of both providers and funders of services. Governments, whether at national, local or some kind of regional level of organization, are often involved in the direct provision of health care services. The extent of provision varies so that in Britain public provision is the dominant method of delivery, whilst in America the service provision role of national government is much less important. Capital investment decisions on the adoption of an innovation by governments, in their role as health service providers, have to be understood within a public policy framework. Considerations such as the scope of government income-generating capacity through trading and taxation and the expected profitability and rate of return on government investment have to be set alongside many other social and political considerations. Government actions also influence the investment decisions of other providers through complicated structures of direct loans, subsidies and grants as well as arrangements through the fiscal system which indirectly affect the cost of investment decisions. Similar structures of support may exist for manufactured goods and commercial services but health, like other kinds of social services, is not regarded as purely a commodity to be bought and sold. Even when market provision is stressed the social dimensions of health care are at least partially acknowledged, including some action to protect those whose health care needs cannot be adequately accommodated by market provision. The justification for government investment or interventions which influence the investment decisions of others through indirect payments and allowances is therefore based upon social as well as economic grounds and incorporates arguments about pro-tecting both individual and community health and well-being.

In any analysis of production there are important distinctions to be made between final and intermediate services and products and also whether the outputs are marketed or non-marketed. Final services involve the provision of services directly to the consumers of those services for their own use. Intermediate ser-vices are equivalent to service products and entail firms employ-ing labour directly, or perhaps more usually through contracting specialist service agencies. These intermediate agencies provide services which are not supplied directly to the end user but are necessary in the production of final services which the consumer receives. Examples of groups which produce intermediate ser-vices would be advertising agencies, management consultancy firms and social services programme evaluation agencies. The other element to be considered is whether services are marketed or non-marketed. Non-marketed services are important in the welfare state, including health care, where it is often thought not desirable for consumers to purchase services directly and it is also difficult to identify the costs to consumers of service provision as there are no equivalents in marketed services against which to make comparisons.

The decision to invest in a health care innovation is influ-enced by the importance of intermediate services in health care production. The era in which health care was encapsulated within the relationship between doctor and patient has long since disappeared. In the home-based service of the nineteenth century the doctor diagnosed and treated the patient. If a drug was required the doctor made up the drug and included its cost in the fee charged. The service transaction involved the doctor, the patient and perhaps some family members. Health services, in both the hospital and the community, now involve a wide range of intermediaries in the relationship between doctor and patient. Diagnosis of the patient's condition commonly entails many tests which may be conducted by workers other than the doctor. These tests require other workers to process and interpret the results. The doctor also relies on the pharmaceutical industry for the generation of new drugs and information about their use and efficacy and on chemists and druggists for dispensing these drugs to their patients. Government usually provides regulatory controls over the introduction of new drugs. Doctors also look to information services from their colleagues and through their professional body and journals in order to assess new technologies including drugs.

This pattern of service, in which those providing direct health care services to consumers rely upon a whole range of intermediate products and services, is firmly established in health care. A particularly important intermediate service is the provision of financial services which assist consumers in the purchasing of health care services. These services have evolved from the sick clubs and friendly societies of the nineteenth century into social insurance schemes in the public sector and third-party commercial insurance in the private sector. The influence of innovations in these mechanisms for funding consumption will be analysed later in this chapter. Decisions to commit capital to technological innovations in health must take into account the complex structure of the health care market and the likely reactions of a wide group of intermediary providers to any decision which is made.

Another factor affecting capital commitment is the anticipated response of labour employed in health care. The influence of medical science through the training and professional socialization of health care workers has encouraged them to search for opportunities to be involved in research on health problems. It appears likely that health workers will wish to adopt new technologies if there is a possibility that such technologies may help those with major health problems. Historically the development of hospitals has been influenced by the demands of health workers to respond to serious illness. Abel–Smith (1964) has described how smallpox epidemics were important in attracting professional and other skilled workers to the new public hospitals in the nineteenth century. In health care as a whole, and hospital services in particular, decisions about technological innovation have been influenced by the need to attract and retain highly trained staff. These workers often seek the most up to date technology with which to apply and develop their work. This worker pressure on hospital investment decisions has been identified as one of the important factors contributing to escalating hospital costs in the 1960s and 1970s (Schroeder and Showstack, 1979, pp. 196–8).

The search for capital to realize organizational innovations has to be considered alongside the capital requirements of other forms of innovation. In America, for-profit health care organizations have become of growing importance since the early 1960s. By 1980 for-profit companies provided about 30 per cent of all hospital beds, just less than the 35 per cent of beds provided by non-profit bodies (Starr, 1982). These for-profit organizations have become increasingly large and more complex incorporating both non-profit and for-profit subsidiaries and they have moved from being located at the city and state level to regional and national operating bases. They offer a wide range of health and related services and have concentrated service organization in large corporate bodies. One of the major reasons for this development has been ascribed to the need for access to large amounts of capital in order to realize innovations in medical technology, and larger organizations tend to have more ready access to such capital markets (Fuchs, 1986, pp. 300–15).

Health care producers will act in a similar manner to other producers in that they will consider the likely response of consumers to service and product innovations before deciding whether to proceed with an innovation. The intimate impact of health care on the individual's physical and mental well-being and upon the 'social body' means that consideration of group and societal values will warrant particular consideration. An example of the impact of cultural values on the adoption of health care innovations is provided by the contraceptive technologies of the pill and the IUD. The knowledge and technologies to introduce both innovations considerably predates their adoption. In part this relates to assessments of the feasibility of the innovations

in terms of their reliability and cost of production but changes
in cultural values and an acceptance and understanding of the
likely social effects of these innovations have also been seen as
central to the producers' eventual decision to adopt and invest
in these technologies (Sidel, 1971, p. 133; Vaughan, 1970).

Labour

Kenwood and Lougheed (1982) suggest that labour supply factors can affect the adoption and diffusion of innovations. This
influence comes about either because the quantity of labour is
high and its cost low, relative to capital, or because the availability of labour and its quality is high and therefore capable of
exploiting new technologies. They also point to the importance
of both geographical and occupational mobility amongst the
labour force if technological innovation is to be promoted and
realized.

What changes have occurred in the size and composition of
the labour force in health care services? The importance of the
health care industry within the economy as a whole in industrial
economies has already been emphasized. In America 1.3 per cent
of the total labour force was employed in health services in 1910
but by 1970 nearly 3 million people were employed comprising
3.8 per cent of the total labour force (Mick, 1981). By 1973 health
comprised the second ranking industrial classification in America
and the employment figures do not include those employed in
the pharmaceutical and medical supply industry (Stoman, 1976,
p. 33). For every 100 patients in American hospitals in 1973
there were 233 full-time equivalent staff employed to provide
health services to these patients. A similar pattern is apparent
in Britain for the higher and lower professional occupational
classes working in health care services. In 1921 0.9 per cent
of the total labour force was employed in these professional
occupations but by 1971 this had risen to 2.4 per cent (Routh,
1980, pp. 13 and 17).

These figures conceal important differences in the growth of
employment within different occupational groups in the health
system. Table 3.1 describes the relative rates of employment
between different occupational groups in health care in America
between 1910 and 1970. In absolute terms the numbers of

Table 3.1 Health care occupations as a percentage of total health
service employment in America

Year	1910	1930	1950	1970
Doctors	30.2	18.6	14.1	9.6
Nurses (Registered)	17.2	34.2	34.1	28.3
Technicians	1.3	5.1	25.6	42.6

Source: Derived from Mick, 1981, p. 108.

doctors, nurses, technologists and technical aides has increased
throughout the sixty-year period but the growth has been more
pronounced amongst registered nurses during the middle of the
period and amongst technologists since the Second World War.
This picture has been replicated in Britain with the numbers
of doctors increasing by just over twofold from 1921 to 1971
whilst the numbers of nurses and other health care workers in the
lower professional classes has increased just under fourfold and
just over fourfold respectively (Routh, 1980). The changes for
professional workers in health care contrast with those in other
industrial and service sectors in the American economy where it
is professional jobs which have increased more rapidly than any
other type of work since 1960. Singelmann and Tienda (1985)
have shown that professional jobs in health care have increased
but they have not increased more quickly than growth in other
types of work especially that of technicians who operate and
maintain the escalating volume of machinery that accompanies
modern medicine. They also argue that the rate of growth in
employment in health care has slowed towards the end of the
1970s. This development is seen as a reflection of changing
economic conditions and the impact of health workers trying
to maintain personal incomes as the number of workers in the
health services increases and the income of consumers and other
sources of funding is constrained.

The question is, what effect has the labour market structure
in health had upon the adoption and diffusion of technological
innovations? The formation of professional associations amongst
doctors, which dated from before the middle of the nineteenth
century in both America and Britain, had a major influence upon
the occupational structure in medicine from the latter part of the
century. Medical education provisions expanded, including the
growth of university-based medical schools, with government

encouraging and promoting these developments. The ideas of medical science were gradually incorporated within the curricula of medical schools: for example, the Flexner Report in 1910 in America emphasized the importance of positivistic science as the basis for medical education and medical practice. The profession gained increasing influence over the entry requirements for access to the profession and in determining the length of training required. This control applied both for people seeking entry within a country and those wishing to enter from outside. These developments mirrored those in other professions such as law and science.

The emergence of specialization amongst physicians has already been noted with the first specialty board being established in America in 1916 (Sidel, 1971, p. 165), and specialization spread beyond the hospital and into general practice during the following fifty years. The work of allied health occupational groups has also reflected the twin moves towards defined entry and training requirements and internal processes of specialization within each occupation. Larkin (1983, p. 3) has described the pattern of labour in health care as an increasingly elaborate hierarchy of occupations in which boundaries between occupations are carefully monitored and controlled and in which workers are at least partially protected from changes in labour market conditions.

There are differing views as to what effect the control over health care work which workers have been able to exert has had upon technological innovation and diffusion in health care. Mannor and Morone (1981) have described the medical profession in America as being innovative in comparison to other occupations and the medical industry as a whole as being characterized by high levels of innovation. This propensity to innovate may be a reflection of professional values which apply in health care. If it is thought technically possible to offer positive help to a patient in any way then that action should be taken. Fuchs (1986) has suggested that there could be wider influences at work connected to both the fascination of the public with technology and the potential personal importance of health care interventions. It is for these reasons that public interest and pressure for technological innovations in health care is particularly high.

Innovation is also viewed as one of the critical ways in which status is achieved in health occupations both within areas of specialist knowledge and in establishing specialties. Innovation is a means by which groups increase their own status either by establishing new areas of activity or by taking over higher status activities from others. These claims to perform certain work and to achieve recognition within the complex of health occupational hierarchies are sanctioned by the various professional organizations. They are also frequently confirmed by government in the form of registration or certification procedures and by employers in both the public and private sectors who are unwilling to offer employment to 'non-certified' labour (Larkin, 1983, p. 5; Schroeder and Showstack, 1979, pp. 180–2).

The ability to impose a uniform but complex pattern of occupational differentiation across the health care industry means that geographical mobility nationally, and to some extent internationally, is achieved for many occupational groups. High levels of mobility would be expected given professional values which emphasize professional advancement and commitment to knowledge generation rather than organizational commitment. High mobility would also be expected given research evidence on general labour turnover. This research indicates that factors such as high educational level, experience of independent working and the kind of role conflict engendered by patient/profession/organization demands would all be indicative of high levels of turnover in an occupational group (see, for example, Mobley, 1982; Mowday *et al.*, 1982). Whilst there may be high levels of geographical mobility in the health labour force, mobility between occupational groups and across specialist interests within occupation groups is likely to be very low. An elaborate occupational hierarchy has evolved in health, in which task boundaries are carefully defined and policed by the relevant occupational groups. These distinctions are also reinforced by employers and the overall result is that there can be little scope for crossing the demarcation boundaries which have been drawn between work performed by different specialties or occupational groups.

There seems to be pressure towards high rates of innovation in health care stemming from professional ideologies, public attitudes and high geographical mobility and at the same time constraints on innovation derived from low levels of occupational mobility. As was previously noted, Kenwood and Lougheed have linked rapid technological innovation with high levels of occupational mobility. Mannor and Morone (1981) indicate a possible explanation for high rates of observed innovation. It may be that health care workers are responsive to innovations in what have been described here as diagnostic and treatment technologies, including the system of individual patient care, but tend to be resistant to innovations in organizational and service delivery technologies. Attempts to change the organization of services, including financing, are most likely to threaten the way in which workers have organized their occupational structures and therefore resistance to these changes would not be unexpected. Overall the attitude towards innovation by health care workers may be partially dependent upon the type of innovation being promoted.

If technological innovation in health care has generally been dynamic, and indeed too rapid for those who blame technological innovation in the 1960s and 1970s as a primary cause of cost escalations in health expenditures, how can high rates of innovation be reconciled with the sustained increase in the size of the labour force which was described earlier? Surely the investment of capital to realize innovations should have led to the substitution of capital for labour? Is the growth in the health labour force generated by similar factors to those which operate in other service activities? That is, is the labour force of lower quality to that in non-service work, working a shorter working week, with a slower rate of technological change and a lower per capita rate of capital investment (Rothwell and Zegveld, 1981, pp. 222–7)? Firstly, whilst discussing factors which affect capital investment decisions in health care, it was noted that the decision is not solely a reflection of economic criteria such as the rate of return and risk factors but of a much more complex web of factors in which the social and political environment play a part. Secondly it appears that the major technological changes in health which have occurred during the last 150 years have seldom provided a simple substitute for labour. The introduction of X-rays for example certainly involved investment in plant and machinery in order to provide this service. However, the innovation also enhanced the diagnostic skills available too the doctor, once he/she was trained in the new technology, and also generated the need for new forms of labour to operate and maintain this new technology. This is typical of most of the major innovations which were identified in Chapter 2. The qualities of existing labour have often been enhanced by an innovation and the labour training associated with the innovation. Innovations have commonly generated new professional or sub-professional groups of labour whose skill is required to provide intermediate services between the doctor and health consumer. Increasingly innovations have created the necessity for technologists and technicians to assist in the operation and maintenance of the machinery involved in an innovation and this has been clearly shown in changes in the size and structure of the health service's labour force. The labour-enhancing nature of many innovations should be taken into account by those who argue that sustained growth in the employment of labour in health care is due to the control which the health occupations have been able to exercise over their own members, their employers and government health policies (see Larkin, 1983).

This debate raises an important question about the capability of innovations in health care to provide options for labour replacement. The traditional mode of health care production was based upon the doctor–patient relationship. The evolution of modern health care is still based upon a personal interaction between doctor and patient even though this interaction is underpinned by a wide range of intermediate services and products. Health care is an extremely complex task and the move towards an industrial model of service production is still quite recent in origin. The option of labour-replacing rather than labour-enhancing innovations may be related to the stage in development of health care as an industrial activity. Another factor which may affect the generation of labour-substituting technologies will be the availability of labour outside the industry. As has already been described health production has gradually been transferred from the household to the formal health care sector. For much of this period, however, formal health care services have been complemented by the care provided by household members, albeit increasingly under the scrutiny of health professionals. Various social and demographic changes since the Second World War are changing the capacity of the household and other sources of informal care to provide these services. The increase in women's rate of participation in the labour force and the demographic pressures of ageing populations in industrially developed countries are the two most prominent factors. In these circumstances the possibilities of shifting labour costs between formal and informal labour sectors in order to reduce production costs becomes less viable. Viewing innovation as at least in part a reflection of demand, one would expect to see more attention to innovations which can substitute for labour whether in the formal health care sector or indeed the informal sector of the household.

TECHNOLOGICAL CHANGE AND CONSUMPTION OF HEALTH CARE

The growth of health care services which are either directly provided or alternatively funded by government is a core element in the emergence of welfare states in developed countries. Consumption of services, such as health care, has been described as one of the means by which social integration is achieved in complex, industrialized and urbanized societies (Flora and Heidenheimer, 1981b). The process of transferring tasks previously performed within the family to service institutions such as the hospital- and community-based health organizations is a part of a series of wider societal changes through which new integrative social mechanisms are created. The manner in which health services are organized and delivered, however, increasingly comes to replicate the forms of production which take place in the industrial realm.

Technological innovations which have occurred outside the specific arena of health care have had important effects on the consumption of health care services and some illustrations of this were briefly described in the previous chapter. Innovations in both personal and public transportation systems and communications systems such as telegraph, telephone, television and facsimile machines have affected the ability of consumers to gain access to health services. This influence is apparent in several changes including the ease of physical access to services, in gaining information about health services and in achieving financial access.

There have always been differences between groups of consumers in their consumption patterns. Smith (1979) notes the clear differences in smallpox treatment between the rich and poor during the nineteenth century. The rich were treated by isolating them from others, controlling their diet and administering quinine and antimonial purges. The poor were required to stay in bed, kept warm and given no alcohol, and no fresh air was allowed into the bedroom. These differences were also apparent in the willingness of patients to try new treatments. Smith notes the willingness of the rich to try vaccination for smallpox whilst the poor were reluctant to try this new method of intervention.

Consumers can also exert some influence over which health issues are viewed as being of particular importance for study and the types of innovations which might be adopted. Verbrugge (1979), for example, has explored the role which middle-class women played in focusing attention upon personal health issues in the mid-nineteenth century and has drawn parallels with the focus of the women's movement in the 1950s and 1960s.

MARKETING INNOVATIONS AND CONSUMPTION

Innovations in the marketing of health care services, especially in the way in which services are paid for, have been of major importance in influencing the level of consumption of health services. For much of the nineteenth century access to a physician's services was confined to the rich who could afford to pay the cost of the service. In America physicians might charge a fee based on the service actually provided or a fixed fee each year to provide health care needed by an individual or family (Starr, 1982). As incomes increased in the latter part of the nineteenth century more people could afford to use doctors' services. This extension was also promoted at this time by the way in which many doctors were willing to make differential charges according to the economic circumstances of their patients and allowed credit by deferring payment.

In Britain collective action through individual contributions to 'sick clubs' and friendly societies began to affect access to health care from the early part of the nineteenth century (Gosden, 1961). Until the 1870s, friendly societies mainly helped members through the payment of sickness benefits and funeral payments. The societies employed the advice of a surgeon, medical officer or apothecary and the supplying of medicines to members also became a common feature of these schemes by the mid-1870s. At this time the early medical aid associations were formed, such as the Manchester Unity Medical Aid Association. These associations employed a full-time medical officer who was expected to practise solely for members of the association and their families. The extension of coverage to all family members became a common component within such schemes. Medical aid associations grew rapidly in the latter part of the century. The idea of a payment to the doctor based upon a fixed sum for each person on their 'list' or 'panel' became an established feature of these schemes and was later incorporated into the national insurance and national health systems. Voluntary sickness funds of a similar type to those in Britain did exist in America during the latter part of the nineteenth century and beginning of the twentieth century but the schemes were less well developed and did not permeate amongst the population to the same extent as they did in Britain.

As was explained in the previous chapter, access to hospitals during the last century was generally based upon the decisions of those who funded the hospitals through subscriptions. Hospitals for much of the century essentially 'stored' the poor and marginal members of society. As the various kinds of technological innovations in diagnosis and treatment, which have been described earlier, were introduced into the hospital the attitude of potential consumers towards hospital treatment gradually changed and access to hospital services was actively sought. The idea that consumption of the hospital service should be based upon payment ran contrary to the established system which had operated in the hospitals. Hospitals run by charitable bodies and public authority hospitals in Britain were, however, criticized in the early part of the twentieth century for treating people without charge who could afford to pay all or part of the cost of treatment (Abel-Smith, 1964, p. 215).

It appears that Britain and America have followed quite divergent routes in the innovations in forms of payment for consumption of health care services which have been introduced in the two countries during the twentieth century.

Britain adopted the general approach of 'social insurance', an innovation whose roots lay in Germany during the 1880s and which diffused widely throughout Europe during the first two decades of the twentieth century (Flora and Heidenheimer, 1981a, chapters 1 and 2). Ritter (1986) says that social insurance in Germany brought together three forms of collective action outside the traditional channels of church, family and voluntary organization. These were first the system of mutual benefit associations which were based in the guilds, corporations and journeyman associations, second the recognition of an employer's obligations to offer protection to employees which had been established in Prussian law since the end of the eighteenth century, and finally the provision of relief for the poor through state and local government institutions.

In Britain similar forms of collective action were in place. Public provision of poor relief was long established through the Poor Laws. There had occurred a dramatic growth in friendly societies', and later trade unions', involvement in the formation of medical care associations which offered their members a means of providing health care for themselves and their families. Concern about working conditions in general, and especially in factories, and the incidence and severity of accidental injuries at work led to a range of factory and workshop legislation during the 1890s. This legislation included the 1897 Workmen's Compensation Act which made employers liable for accidents in the workplace and required them to insure against such events and to compensate workers irrespective of the cause of the accident. The coverage of this legislation was subsequently extended in 1906.

The 1911 National Health Insurance Act made general medical services available to manual workers and other employees whose income was less than £160 per annum. The scheme was based upon contributions to an approved medical association by the worker, the employer and the state. The new system went some way towards improving access to health care, but coverage under the scheme was limited because dependents and those not in paid work were not included and hospital and specialist care was also excluded.

Private health insurance through third parties or by doctors or hospitals did not become widely established in Britain during the early part of the twentieth century. This has been attributed to the level of health care charges relative to the incomes of middle- and upper-class patients at this time (Watkin, 1978, p. 10) which meant that many people could afford to pay doctors' bills out of their regular incomes. Hospital care was still provided free of charge to most low-income patients on a means-tested basis.

During the 1920s and 1930s, as the economic depression affected incomes, provident schemes which were often run by hospitals themselves provided access to inpatient and outpatient hospital care and specialist services but not to general practitioner services (Honigsbaum, 1979). Workers made regular contributions to these funds and in return they were not required to pay charges for hospital services and the money raised by contributions was distributed between the voluntary hospitals in the local geographical area. By the beginning of the Second World War about half the population were covered by these types of contributory schemes (Watkin, 1978). Despite the growing use of contributory schemes the financial viability of many voluntary hospitals was under threat and financial support by government became increasingly important to the continued survival of many hospitals. The full realization of the social insurance approach to health care in Britain came about in 1948 with the creation of the National Health Service which established accesss to general practitioner, specialist and hospital care for the whole population funded through compulsory contributions from employed people, employers and the state.

The picture of innovations in consumption in America is rather different. Collective action by consumers to provide life insurance and financial support during illness did develop through consumer clubs from the beginning of the nineteenth century (Abel-Smith, 1976, pp. 9–10; Starr, 1982, p. 205). The coverage and scope of these groups was not as great as their counterparts in Britain and the American Medical Association was implacably opposed to their operation. Some employers, in activities such as railroads and mining, made direct provision of emergency medical care to their employees. There was a move towards extending employer provision from an emergency basis to a much wider concern for general employee health. These ideas were realized in actions to improve working conditions for employees and Starr (1982, p. 200) has linked these actions to promote industrial hygiene with the ideas of scientific management associated with Frederick Taylor. Employer control over the choice of doctor and use of medical care was resisted by the American Federation of Labor. The extent of employer provision reached a peak in the 1920s but was confined to certain industries and geographical areas. The onset of the major depression of the 1920s and 1930s severely affected the level of direct employer provision.

From 1890 to 1930 some employers acted through third parties or in association with each other to create mutual funds. In parts of the logging, mining and railroad industries workers themselves paid into mutual funds which were also financially supported by the employer. Stock and mutual companies offered insurance policies which provided for a continuation of family income in the event of illness or accident (Richardson, 1945, p. 17).

Some hospitals developed plans in which specified facilities were made available to a subscriber in return for a direct payment. These single-hospital plans were initially few in number and offered varied levels of services and financial security. The financial problems which were engendered by the depression for hospitals in Britain also threatened the financial viability of hospitals in America. The transformation in consumption of hospital services came about through the hospitals themselves as they developed and promoted voluntary insurance in a scheme called 'Blue Cross'. Blue Cross was developed from an initial innovation which had begun at the Baylor University Hospital in Dallas in 1929 which offered about 1,250 school teachers up to twenty-one days of hospital care each year for a payment of $6 for each person (Law, 1974). Other hospitals and groups of hospitals adopted the innovation, for example in Sacramento in 1932 and Essex, New Jersey, in 1933. Some plans allowed subscribers to be treated in any one of a group of hospitals in a city or region. The American Hospital Association (AHA) approved the principle of insurance coverage of hospital care in 1933 and the American College of Surgeons followed suit in 1934. The professional and legal framework under which the schemes were to operate was developed by the AMA which laid down a series of principles for the plans and guidelines for enabling legislation which was required to be passed through each state legislature. New York pioneered enabling legislation in 1934 and by 1945 similar legislation had been passed in thirty-five states. The number of Blue Cross plans expanded rapidly from twenty-three in 1933 to seventy-one by 1942 (Richardson, 1945, p. 36) and by 1945 about 19 million people were subscribers to Blue Cross plans (Starr, 1982, p. 311).

There were attempts to replicate Blue Cross by introducing similar prepayment schemes for general practitioner services in the late 1920s and early 1930s. These proposals were opposed by the AHA who had hoped that with the establishment of Blue Cross more people would then be able to pay fees for general practitioner services at the point of service. Increasing activity by private insurers contributed to a growing public acceptance of prepayment schemes for general medical services and several plans developed in California and Michigan in 1939. Gradually these plans became more widely adopted and became known as 'Blue Shield'. By 1942/3 the AHA was formally prepared to accept the development of Blue Shield plans and in 1945 about 2 million people subscribed to these plans (Starr, 1982, p. 311). Blue Cross and Blue Shield offered similar coverage to that available through social insurance schemes in other countries in the sense that they accepted all members of the community irrespective of age or risk – they were what Abel-Smith (1976, p. 21) has referred to as 'community-related' plans.

Private insurers in America began to make substantial inroads into the health market in the early 1940s offering premium payments related to individual risk. Private insurance schemes were also supported by employers who were prepared to pay premiums for employees as a way of attracting scarce labour and by unions who sought health care coverage from employers for their members. In 1946 only just over half a million workers were covered by union-negotiated plans, but from 1948 onwards unions became more active in seeking to negotiate health coverage in their awards and by 1954 12 million workers and 17 million dependants were covered. The diffusion of insurance, especially through hospital plans, has been extensive – in 1945 a quarter of the population had insurance, 14.8 per cent under Blue Cross and 8.2 per cent with commercial insurers, and by 1975 84.2 per cent of the population were insured, 40.9 per cent with Blue Cross and 47.1 per cent with commercial insurers (Feldstein, 1979, table 7.1, p. 136). The contribution of insurance to private health care payments has also increased dramatically – in 1955 insurance accounted for 18.2 per cent of payments but by 1976 it was 38.9 per cent (Feldstein, 1979, table 3.3, p. 33).

Attempts to introduce some form of social insurance in America to cover health care services have a long history. The American Federation of Labor was particularly active in lobbying for change in the period from 1910 to 1920. Most explanations for why this pressure for innovation in the consumption of health care services was not successful stress two major elements. First, the infrastructure required for a social insurance scheme was not available at this time despite the fact that similar innovations were being introduced throughout Europe. The structures of government activity and intervention at federal and state level were not as long established or as extensive as their European counterparts. This observation applied similarly to other types of collective action, through groups of workers in unions and friendly societies, for example. Second was the impact of major differences in both the cultural values and social and political environments between America and Europe. These differences included the lack of a major perceived threat from organized labour in America, the related absence of a move towards developing political socialism and finally the emphasis in America upon individual liberalism and minimal government.

Polsky (1984, pp. 153–63) has described the eventual introduction of health insurance for the aged through Medicare over fifty years after the initial campaign of the Federation of Labor as an example of what he refers to as an 'incubated' innovation. In these kinds of policy areas there is usually little agreement over the exact nature of the problem being addressed. The issue is taken up by many diverse groups in different forms and conflict is generated about the issues both at an ideological and policy level. The capacity to focus the policy environment upon the issue and crystallize a concrete policy innovation takes a considerable period of time.

In America there was a growth in government involvement in the funding of research and training and in assisting hospital construction in the postwar period, but direct action to assist consumption did not emerge until the 1960s. The Kerr–Mills Bill allowed federal assistance to states through grants towards the cost of providing medical care to those amongst the aged who were judged to be financially unable to meet their own health needs (Stevens and Stevens, 1974). Some states responded to this initiative but others could not, or would not, pay their part of the cost of the scheme. In 1965 new legislation was passed which provided for compulsory hospital insurance for the aged, subsidization of voluntary insurance to cover fees for general practitioner services and improved help, although still means-tested, for medical care of the poor.

This major innovation has contributed to a dramatic change in the balance of funding of health care consumption. In 1955 almost three-quarters of expenditure on medical care was financed through private payments, and of the quarter financed by public payments 56 per cent came from state and local government payments and 44 per cent from federal sources. In 1976 only 57.3 per cent of expenditure came from private payments and 42.7 per cent from public payments and nearly 68 per cent of this came from federal payments (Feldstein, 1979, p. 33). These figures underestimate federal contributions to medical care expenditure as they do not include tax forgone through allowances to individuals and companies against health care insurance premiums. The OECD (1985a) has estimated these tax expenditures at just over $24 billion in 1983.

Marketing innovations in both private and public sectors have had an important influence upon the pattern of consumption of health care in both Britain and America. In each country there are some common features in the changes in consumption. Innovations have been introduced which have extended the consumption of health care services throughout the popula-tions of both countries so that all, or at least the vast major-ity, of the population have access to health services. The cost of consumption is borne by a combination of the individ-ual consumer, employers of labour and government through the generation and application of tax funds whether generated by national or local units of government. Differences in the balance between the three funders of consumption in Britain and America have tended to diminish over time. Public funding, which has in any case historically been underestimated in America because of the exclusion of fiscal welfare measures from the expenditure figures, has increased in importance in America during the last twenty to thirty years. Conversely private funding through individual consumer and employer payments has become of increasing importance in the British health system. There remains a major difference in the technological base of consumption in that the American system is mainly based upon individual insurance principles in which coverage and cost is calculated in accordance with the calculation of individual risk, whilst the British system, through publicly organized social insurance, broadly provides coverage for all irrespective of risk. The cost to the individual in the British system will reflect the incidence of the personal taxation system including compulsory national insurance contributions. This difference between the American and British health systems has narrowed as publicly financed coverage of high-risk groups has increased in America and the contribution of private-insurance-backed health care has increased in Britain.

'SOCIAL INNOVATION' AND FUTURE HEALTH CARE PRODUCTION AND CONSUMPTION

Before considering future changes in the way health care is produced and consumed it is necessary to consider a further dimension in our conceptual approach to technological change. The various explanations of technical and social invention and innovation which have been described until this point assume that the impetus for change comes from a complex mix of actions from the various parties to the production of goods and services with the final individual consumer also having an influence. Gershuny (1983a; 1983b; 1984; 1985; Gershuny and Miles, 1983) and his colleagues at the Science Policy Research Unit at Sussex University have developed an explanation of technological change which acknowledges the role of the household in influencing technological change. The household, rather than the individual *per se*, is at the centre of consumption of goods and services, even though economists seldom appear to recognize this. Each household has a range of needs which it seeks to meet over time such as transport, communication, accommodation, domestic services, food, leisure and so on. How these requirements are met Gershuny refers to as the 'mode of provision' and innovation occurs when there are changes in this mode. Social innovation in this sense influences the division of time between the paid and unpaid work of household members as they seek to meet household needs.

Whilst the household is the focal point for the consumption of goods and services it is extremely important to recognize its position relative to production. Goods and services can be bought from outside the household but they can also be produced by household members or produced through transactions in informal channels such as the 'black' economy or communal exchange. Gershuny's emphasis upon the household has some similarities with aspects of Rein's (1983, chapter 2) analysis of the welfare state. Rein sees each household as defining a unique set of claims against different systems of resources including the private and public systems of producing goods and services. Both Gershuny and Rein are demonstrating that we cannot treat the household as a passive or merely responsive unit to changes in economic and political systems. Households are constantly assessing changes in the relative prices of goods and services and alternative modes of producing them and social innovations in those modes.

The decisions which households make have major implications for the system of production outside the household. Whilst Gershuny (1983a, chapters 2 and 3) accepts the proposition put forward by the economist Fred Hirsch that as households become better off they tend to consume more luxury or, as Hirsch describes them, positional goods and services attracted partially by their scarcity, he warns about the limitations of the associated proposition that industrial development will inevitably lead towards the creation of a service based economy. Gershuny, like Boudon (1986), demonstrates the limitations of such an approach which rests upon comparing two points in time and seeking to explain change on the basis of a simple comparison. He illustrates this point by looking at the services enjoyed by well-off households in the nineteenth and early twentieth centuries. The well off employed domestic servants, were transported in carriages and trains and went to concerts and the theatre. When the poor became better off they did not meet those needs in the same way but rather met them through domestic machinery and their own labour in the house, driving their personal transport in the form of the motor car and accessing entertainment in their own homes through television and video. There are major innovations in the mode of production involved here which illustrate the capacity for manufactured products combined with domestic labour to substitute for expensive services within the domestic household. Gershuny (1983a, p. 51) has described the traditional mode of service provision as being relatively labour-intensive, usually involving face-to-face interaction with quite low fixed costs but high marginal costs. In these circumstances there are incentives to change the mode of provision through the production of material goods which can displace expensive labour and the provision of labour from within the household or informal economy, thereby emphasizing self-service rather than direct servicing. These changes within the household may interact in many ways with the introduction of innovations in the service sector and may be of special significance in the pattern of future innovation in social services, including health care.

Health care production has gradually been transferred from a household base to the equivalent of a factory base in the form of increasingly large, complex and centralized institutions such as the hospital, group practice or health maintenance organization. Examples of this transfer in the locus of production were described earlier in this chapter. Radical innovations in health care were classified and identified in Chapter 2. An examination of the impact of these innovations upon the production of services and the factors of production in health care indicated that these innovations have frequently not provided a substitute for labour but have rather been 'labour enhancing' and have generated increasing demands for new labour skills. This impact upon the demand for labour skills has been reflected in the growth and composition of the health care labour force in both America and Britain.

There may be particular reasons why capital or commodity substitution in health care appears to have been relatively minor in scope. Blackburn *et al.* (1985, pp. 178–80) have suggested that the extensiveness of professional work and control which professional associations exert over that work in social services will act as a brake upon innovations which might threaten substitution for labour. This view is shared by many commentators on health issues who would cite firstly the selective adoption of innovations which may serve the interests of professional workers rather than necessarily the interests of consumers or funders, and secondly the general effects of labour force rigidities which they believe reflect the power of professional hierarchies within health care services.

There are other possible reasons why labour substitution does not appear to have been a major influence in the health sector. One explanation is that the level of technological development in health care has been such that capital substitution in the complex tasks involved has not been possible. The lack of labour substitution is therefore merely a manifestation of a limited technological base. Another possible explanation is that it is a limitation implied by government provision and funding of health services in industrially develloped countries. Health care is usually at least partially publicly funded because of the claimed social effects associated with consumption and lack of consumption. The need for social control over consumption is much easier to achieve in a large publicly owned or controlled institution such as a hospital rather than in the household (Blackburn *et al.*, 1985).

Adopting Gershuny's ideas about 'innovation in provision', households can be viewed as having a range of needs for products and services including health, education and housing. These are all services in which public provision or funding play an important role in modern industrial economies. The technologies, including the organizational technologies, available to households to satisfy household needs change over time. The means which a household uses to meet its needs, its 'mode of provision', will change as alternative modes are assessed. It is these changes in the mode of provision within households and amongst informal producers within the community, as well as at a societal level, which Gershuny refers to as 'social innovation'. Health care services as they have developed outside the household conform to what Gershuny refers to as the traditional mode of provision in that they are labour-intensive and usually involve face-to-face contact. Capital investment has been concentrated in buildings and is therefore expected to last for a long period of time. Fixed costs are low but marginal costs are high and predominantly reflect labour costs. These are not the conditions under which high rates of social innovation might be expected to occur.

Both Gershuny and Blackburn have been interested in describing changes in social innovation and in particular how changes have occurred over time and between different groups in society. Entertainment which was enjoyed by the wealthy outside the home in the form of theatre, ballet, opera and so on was transformed for access to the majority of the population by innovations such as television, gramophone and video into home-based entertainment once the equipment necessary for these innovations was available at a price which was within the reach of households. Two processes are involved: first, the externalization of service labour in that users of services are provided with the means of providing at least part of those services themselves often in their own homes, and, second, restructuring consumption by altering the range of goods and services available.

The institutional arrangements under which health care services are provided are not static. Despite this the basic infrastructure of hospital-dominated care and community-based services in centres containing general practitioners and groups of other health care workers is the institutional system which has evolved and been maintained since the late nineteenth century. This system transferred health from household production to institutional production and was established partly by pointing to the inadequacies and dangers of household-based production of health. The public sanctioning and control of health care, alongside other social services, has been particularly apparent during the last fifty years in most OECD countries. The public institutionalization of health services in this way may have contributed to a labour-intensive and increasingly expensive health service given the rise in the relative costs of labour in the postwar period.

Gershuny (1983a, p. 51) says that there are three ways in which labour requirements of a service might be reduced: first, through the mechanization of physical work performed by labour, second, by automation of the tasks themselves, and finally through the incorporation of the knowledge and skills of service workers in an alternative form. Health services entail the most intimate forms of personal services to the bodies and minds of consumers. Whilst there may be scope for mechanization of indirect services which support patient care it is hard to see, given present technologies, any substantial mechanization of patient services. Automation has occurred especially in recent decades with innovations like kidney dialysis machines, body scanners and general patient care monitoring systems. These kinds of developments have been made possible by innovations in areas such as electronics. These systems have in some cases substituted for one form of labour but frequently require the utilization of other forms of labour to maintain and monitor the machines themselves.

The incorporation of medical knowledge in computer software packages which can be linked to diagnostic and monitoring machinery represents an important future opportunity for reducing labour requirements. It offers the possibility of servicing a given group of people with less labour. There are more dramatic possibilities in terms of the mode of production which might be possible given the combination of these kinds of innovations with the development of other products and services and the infrastructure necessary for these innovations. Radical innovations in communication technologies may transform the capacity of households to receive and transmit information with the external environment. The availability of personal computer technology within households and the linkage of these innovations to those in the telecommunications industry such as microwave communication techniques might make it possible to see households once again in a position to produce aspects of health care for their members which they cannot presently provide.

Households have not ceased to produce health care in modern health care systems. Self-care, the care of family members through mutual aid and the use of patent medicines and other remedies, obviously still make a substantial contribution to personal health production. The formalization and professionalization of health care has concentrated what is regarded as legitimate knowledge in the formal health care system and its workers. The incorporation of that knowledge in packages such as computer-aided self-diagnostic programmes, monitoring machines for assessing the condition of those with chronic long-term illness and computer linkages between consumers and their carers and health professionals offer the prospect of changes in the mode of production. Such changes in the mode of production would affect the relationship between health workers and consumers and the balance between labour and capital inputs in health care production. The infrastructure necessary for such changes to take place will not come about through health care concerns alone but rather as a consequence of wider changes in which households' communication and information systems are being transformed.

4 Political Innovation and Health Care

The contribution which governments make to the production of health care has to be understood against the much wider picture of government action which influences the general production of goods and services within an economy. The welfare states which have evolved in the Western industrial countries during the course of the last century have involved government actions to meet the health care needs of their populations. Those actions have taken many forms including the direct provision of health care services by the state, mechanisms to fund consumers to gain access to services and indirect actions which affect other producers. The state both constructs and mediates the environment in which producers, funders and consumers of health care operate through mechanisms such as subsidies, grants, taxes and legal requirements. As Bice (1981, p. 43) implies, all changes in public services and public policies represent forms of innovation. Government policy prescriptions alter the way health care services are organized and delivered and therefore represent an important source of innovations which must be incorporated into an analysis of technological innovation in health care.

DIRECT PUBLIC PROVISION AND FUNDING

The objective here is to describe some of the main innovations in direct provision and funding of health care in Britain and America and to outline the rather different experiences in the two countries in this regard. The focus is narrowly upon policy changes as technological innovations rather than the much wider set of parameters in which public policy decisions are grounded.

However, as for the analysis of all policy it is helpful to ask the question, who is meant to benefit from innovations in the public provisions – the individual, his or her family, the service provider or the community as a whole?

Britain

The history of the development of government provision of health care in Britain has been closely related to the institutional arrangements of the Poor Laws. Central government made grants to local government authorities and acting through boards of guardians in each local district the system of workhouses and financial relief was organized. A district medical officer was appointed for each district who made home visits or visits to sick wards or dispensaries within the workhouse. The standard of the service provided was usually very low. From the 1860s onwards there was a limited development of public hospitals under the auspices of the Metropolitan Asylums Board through which care was provided for those with infectious diseases who were commonly excluded from admission to voluntary hospitals and workhouse dispensaries. The state was also active in seeking to ensure vaccination against smallpox within the community through several pieces of legislation from 1840 to 1871. The 1853 Act required that all infants under three months of age must be vaccinated. The system was administered under the Poor Law with vouchers being provided to poor families to be exchanged for vaccination by any doctor (Smith, 1979, p. 161). Public provision of health care during this period was mostly confined to a small and clearly identifiable section of the community. Health care provision was part of a wider system of government action through which it was thought that community well-being was promoted through closely controlling the poor.

During the nineteenth century the population of Britain was transformed from a rural-based population to an urban population. In 1801 only 20 per cent of the population in England and Wales lived in towns but by 1911 about 80 per cent were town dwellers (Wohl, 1983). The emergence of the sanitary reform movement and its objectives and achievements has already been described. The 1848 Public Health Act enabled local government authorities to take over the responsibility for water supply from private companies. Despite the heavy capital cost involved in doing so about one-third of water supply provision passed to local authorities by 1871. The 1872 Public Health Act placed an obligation upon local authorities to provide water supplies. By the turn of the century about two-thirds of local authorities had met this obligation. Central government provided loans through the Local Government Board for work associated with the provision of water supplies and loans rose sharply during the 1870s and again in the 1890s (Wohl, 1983, p. 162).

Alongside improvements in water supply were changes in waste disposal techniques. These changes included the replacement of cesspools for the homes of the poor with the pan-and-pail dry-conservancy method in the late 1860s and 1870s. Improvements in water supply allowed the realization of the water closet technology which had been patented by Bramah in 1778. Central and local government action in these areas of health involved provisions which individuals were unlikely to make for themselves and which private providers were unlikely to provide at a cost low enough to ensure universal consumption. Consumption throughout the population benefited the population as a whole as well as individuals, and public health provision was seen as a necessary step to achieve the realization of these community benefits. Public provision encouraged the adoption of technological innovations in the area of water and waste engineering and also enabled innovations such as the water closet to be adopted within private households.

Government involvement in the direct provision of health services increased during the latter part of the nineteenth century with the direct employment of doctors, not just in Poor Law institutions, but also for work in prisons, police and ports. From the beginning of the twentieth century demand for health services was increasing partly in response to the possibilities offered by medical technology and the changing public perception of that technology (Hollingsworth, 1986, p. 19). However, the combination of increasing public demand and increasing costs associated with new technologies meant that many friendly societies were facing financial difficulties. The 1911 National Health Insurance Act was a major policy innovation through which government accepted a financial responsibility for assisting workers on limited incomes to maintain their incomes during sickness and to have access to health services from a general practitioner. The insurance scheme was based upon workers paying four pence a week, employers three pence and the state two pence. This scheme can be viewed as consistent with the general development of social insurance which was emerging within Europe from the late nineteenth century. It differed however from many of its European counterparts with its requirement for compulsory contributions from the three parties. The government achieved a skilful reconciliation of the interests of several groups in this scheme. Medical benefits were administered by local insurance committees which were structured in such a way as to include representatives of the main interest groups. Similarly cash benefits were paid through approved societies including insurance companies, friendly societies and trade unions. General practitioners were amenable to payment being based upon the number of patients on their lists. They also obtained government agreement to the principle that either the doctor or patient could refuse treatment. The structure created by the 1911 Act encouraged the growth of general practice and the system of insurance-backed payment enhanced the incomes of many general practitioners.

The organizational structure of government activity in health provision was strengthened by the creation of the Ministry of Health in 1918. Alongside the growth of the institutional framework of health services at central government level, local government authorities had gradually been absorbing the facilities and responsibilities which had previously been controlled by the boards of guardians under the Poor Law. The move towards greater centralization and complexity in the organization of publicly provided health services was part of the general growth of government which had been taking place since the middle of the nineteenth century, and which had been apparent in health care since the 1848 Public Health Act. Roberts accurately describes this process when he says that: 'The larger the government grew the more it found to reform. An enlarged bureaucracy, in short, tended to further its own growth' (1969, p. 72).

During the 1920s and 1930s the voluntary hospitals again found themselves facing the twin pressures of demand for investment in a wide range of new and improved technologies in surgical and diagnostic techniques and an escalating consumer demand encouraged by such developments in technology. These demands placed the financial viability of many voluntary hospitals in jeopardy at a time when the standards of public hospital provision had much improved. The history of the public hospitals was grounded in the Poor Law and in general they were overcrowded, had poorer physical conditions and fewer staff than other hospitals. They were also slower to adopt new technologies than the voluntary hospitals. The interwar period saw public hospitals offer better physical conditions and staffing than in the past and they demonstrated an increasing awareness of the potential value of new technologies.

There were many concerns expressed at this time about the overall effectiveness of the health care system. The 1911 National Insurance Act had improved access to general medical services but access to hospital and specialist services was generally excluded. Only about one-third of the population was covered by the Act and in particular dependants of those insured under the Act were not covered. There were known to be wide variations in the standard and availability of services in different parts of the country, including the distribution of general practitioner services. The diversity and large number of providers in the private and public sectors also led to worries about the overall organizational coherence of the service.

The 1946 National Health Services Act sought to address these issues and represented a major political innovation in changing the organizational technology of the British health care system. The idea of compulsory insurance for general medical services based upon contributions from workers, employers and the state was extended to cover the entire population. The payment of capitation to doctors and the choice for both doctors and patients to refuse treatment were retained. The scheme was administered by local executive councils. Doctors' incomes were bolstered by the extension of the scheme just as they had been by the 1911 Act, but general practitioners remained isolated from specialist and research services in hospitals and research centres and therefore from direct experience of the changes in technology which were centred on hospital medicine. The Act made dramatic changes in the hospital sector with the nationalization of nearly all hospitals and the opening up of hospital treatment to all the population without direct charges for care.

Organizationally the country was divided into regions with each region being affiliated to a university with a medical school. The regions were administered by regional hospital boards and each hospital had a hospital management committee. Local government authorities retained responsibility for preventive and environmental health services such as health and safety in the workplace and domiciliary services for mothers and infants. This basic organizational structure was to remain in place until 1974 when the three strands of hospital, preventive and community medicine were brought within a structure of comprehensive control under regional and area bodies. The 1946 Act established a health care system in Britain in which the vast majority of care was provided by and funded through the state. There was universal access to free hospital and general practitioner services including free pharmaceutical services.

America

The role of government in the direct provision and funding of health care has been of much less importance to the development of health care in America than in Britain. Public hospital provision existed in America from about the middle of the nineteenth century. Like their British counterparts they provided care for the poor and those who were viewed as a danger to the rest of the community. Local government in towns and counties raised funds to build the hospitals, but once built the expectation was that income generated from fees would be sufficient to cover operating costs. In the cities the funding of large public hospitals was based on the expectation that hospitals would be a charge on local taxes for both their running and foundation costs. The standard of care was poor, physical conditions bad and overcrowding common and the primary purpose of the city hospital was to control the indigent and dangerous.

As in Britain the second half of the nineteenth century saw major developments in public health measures, especially in water supply and waste disposal. These innovations were realized through local government actions although problems associated with the impact of waste disposal schemes adopted by one area upon the water supply of another contributed towards the creation of larger units of administrative and political responsibility at the urban and inter-municipal and inter-state levels (Tarr *et al.*, 1984). At a national level there were moves towards a national agency in the health area with the formation of a National Board of Health in 1879 and the formation of the Public Health Service in 1912.

Major innovations in federal responsibilities for health care provision have occurred since the Second World War. The Hill/Burton legislation of 1948 led to considerable federal funding for the building of medical research centres and the funding of research. The introduction of Medicare and Medicaid in 1965 represented major federal initiatives in direct provision. Medicaid ensured increased federal support for means-tested health care for the poor which was provided by state governments, and Medicare introduced compulsory health care insurance cover for the aged. Government action to ensure access to health care for a section of the population through Medicare occurred over fifty years after similar action for workers in Britain. Whilst this action does represent a move towards direct public action to fund the consumption of health care services there is no evidence that the federal government will also move to direct provision of health care services. In America a great deal of the influence of the federal government on health care comes through indirect action.

INDIRECT ACTION BY GOVERNMENT

Rein (1983, chapter 1) has described a system for classifying the roles which government can adopt in its relationship to the welfare activities undertaken by private sector firms. These roles are mandating, regulating, supporting and stimulating.

1   Regulating – a critical function which governments play is in defining the rules within which social, political and economic relations are conducted. The state has played an important part in welfare activities through seeking to protect individuals within society in their roles as workers and consumers. In the context of health, governments

commonly set standards for activities which affect the health of individuals and communities. Examples of such regulatory activity are found in occupational health and safety legislation and in the identification of minimum safety standards for the food and drink which we consume. The history of welfare state development has been closely linked to government regulation of private providers of social services. These regulations have often been a response by government to public concern over allegations of abuse and ill-treatment of social service recipients; the history of institutional care for the mentally ill in both America and Britain, for example, vividly illustrates this interaction between public concern and government regulation (Armour, 1981; Jones, 1972).

2   Mandating – government, whether at national, regional or local government level, may pass legislation which requires private sector firms to contribute towards, or implement, policies specified by the state. In Britain compulsory national insurance payments by employers is an example of employers being mandated to contribute towards a range of publicly provided social services. The cost of meeting the requirements of government may be fully or partly offset by financial payments by government or firms may be left to meet the costs themselves. If the costs are borne by the firm then these costs may be passed on to others in the production of goods and services including the final consumer.

3   Supporting – financial support by government at various levels can be used to keep private sector providers operating even when those operations are no longer financially viable. Actions of this type have been particularly visible when a major producer of goods or services has been involved and the employment of large numbers of people threatened.

4   Stimulating – government may seek to either encourage or discourage occupational welfare services from employers and private sector providers of social services through financial payments of some kind. These payments may be channelled directly through grants and subsidies or indirectly, for example, through rebates on tax liability or by forgoing tax levies on certain forms of expenditure.

These techniques can be used to encourage individuals to use private sector provision as well as to encourage private providers themselves. They can also be used as a discriminatory mechanism to favour certain types of provision or particular providers rather than others. The threat of withdrawal of these kinds of financial supports can be used as a powerful disincentive to any action of which the government disapproves.

Rein's framework needs some modification for analysing the indirect role which the state plays in relation to private health care provision. First the organizational environment in health care is more complicated than a simple private/public division or a producer/distributor/retailer structure. The importance of the production of intermediate goods and services which may be either marketed or non-marketed means that government, at various levels, confronts an extremely complex environment in which the impact of government actions on the total structure is difficult to predict and describe. Second, in countries such as Britain where government is a major direct provider of health care, there has been in recent years the emergence of contracting or competitiive tendering of services to private firms. This type of contracting has included not just support services such as hospital cleaning and laundering but also the contracting of medical services themselves. Contracting ought therefore to be added to Rein's list of government actions in relation to private sector welfare activities. Third, many workers in health care, especially doctors, are in effect self-employed private sector providers. This is most obviously true in America but also in Britain where the history of general practitioner services in a sense represents an early form of contracting by the state in that doctors contracted to provide general medical services to a defined number of people in return for an annual payment per person. Similarly in British hospitals doctors can work as employed staff on the one hand and self-employed workers in private practice on the other. An understanding of government actions towards private provision of health care must incorporate the interaction of government and a health care labour force which straddles the boundaries between private and public forms of service production.

Using the framework outlined above we are now in a position to assess the possible effects of government activity upon technological innovation in health care in the private sector and the implications of this for public provision.

The impact of the regulatory activity of the state on technological innovation has been widely debated especially in relation to the pharmaceutical industry. In America the 1906 Pure Food and Drug Act was a federal response to public concern about the possible harmful effects of patent medicines which had been highlighted by newspapers combined with pressure from the American Medical Association (Starr, 1982, p. 129). Many of the larger pharmaceutical producers supported federal action and the introduction of regulations has been described as having been a contributing factor in the formation of the American Pharmaceutical Manufacturers Association. Government regulation was therefore itself a factor in stimulating organizational innovations in the industry. Regulation protected the interests of established producers by making entry into the industry more difficult to achieve and it also tended to encourage mergers and takeovers amongst established firms (Liebenau, 1987, pp. 79–81).

Further regulation of the industry has occurred during the twentieth century with the 1938 Food, Drug and Cosmetic Act and the Kefauver-Harris amendments to this Act in 1962. The 1938 Act followed the deaths of over a hundred children and required that new drugs must be approved by the Food and Drug Administration and shown to be safe before being introduced. This innovation came at the threshold of the surge of pharmaceutical innovations such as the antibiotic and sulpha drugs. The 1938 Act also distinguished between ethical drugs which required a doctor's prescription and proprietary drugs which could be bought from the druggist. This separation subsequently influenced the relationship between the pharmaceutical companies and doctors, who controlled prescribing of ethical drugs, and this relationship has affected the adoption and diffusion of new drugs. In America drug companies spend about 10 per cent of their total budget on promotional activity much of it aimed at doctors. In 1962 amendments to the 1938 Act were made which required that new drugs must be shown to be effective, and not merely safe for public use, before they could be introduced and this entailed federal overseeing of the clinical process of drug development and testing (Grabowski and Vernon, 1982).

In Chapter 2 some of the arguments concerning the impact of government regulation upon product innovation and diffusion in the pharmaceutical industry were described. It has been claimed that safety controls are too stringent and that price-restraint mechanisms and controls over advertising too severe. These kind of controls are said to have delayed the introduction of new and effective drugs into the American market by overseas producers. The regulatory environment is seen by some as creating the possible transfer of pharmaceutical production and research facilities out of a closely regulated country into a location where the controls are less pervasive (Brada, 1980). Clearly the regulatory environment which a government insti-gates will be one of the factors which affects the decision of pharmaceutical companies as to whether to pursue and adopt a particular innovation. Such regulations impinge upon the length of product development, likely rate of return and the risk involved in committing investment to the innovation. There are of course many other factors which will also to be taken into account.

The mechanisms through which regulatory controls operate and the total structure of the health industry will also influence decisions. Hollingsworth (1986, pp. 171–5) has suggested that Britain is more likely than America to adopt expensive but effective drugs that are demanded by many different sections of the community. It is said that the smaller number of providers and the important role of the state in direct provision in Britain has led to less rigid regulation. A new drug can be introduced and its value more easily monitored in a centralized system as the information which is generated is more accessible to the state administrative structures. In an environment in which provision is spread through many diverse producers this kind of ongoing monitoring is much more difficult to achieve and therefore much tighter controls over the decision to allow drug usage may be necessary. Britain has also made use of voluntary agreements to control private health care actors such as the pharmaceutical companies. The initiation of the National Health Service coin-cided with the dramatic growth in drug innovations and there was concern about the likely increasing costs of pharmaceutical products. A voluntary price regulation scheme between the pharmaceutical manufacturers and the state was formulated in 1957 and extended to cover all branded ethical products in 1972. This use of negotiated voluntary agreements, albeit backed by statutory controls to deal with breaches of the agreement, has featured in the interaction between government and private sector participants in the British health care system.

Government regulation of the training and practice framework within which professional health care workers operate has long been a feature of health care systems. In Britain, for instance, the 1858 Medical Act identified the legislative framework for the organizational structure of the medical profession (Woodward, 1984, p. 69). Professional bodies, especially amongst doctors, represent some of the strongest and most influential occupational groups in the labour force. Their position has often been facilitated by government encouragement of their associations and government protection from competition from practitioners of alternative forms of health care. Governments have in many ways delegated their regulatory powers to associations of professional health care workers. This delegation has included controls over training and certification and the acceptance of the validity of peer supervision as a means of monitoring and controlling poor standards of medical research and practice. As has been described earlier the broad acceptance that science should be the basis of medicine has permeated the health professions. This influence has been apparent in the approach of health care professions to training, research, career advancement and the organizational structuring of the professions. The readiness of workers to adopt technological innovations, at least certain types of innovation, was described in the previous chapter. The more a government delegates control over professional workers to professional associations, the more likely it would appear to be that innovations in diagnostic and treatment technologies, which are viewed within the professions as scientifically advanced, will be readily adopted by workers.

The analysis and critique of professional power in many areas of social life including medicine, and concern at escalating private and public costs of health care in the 1960s and 1970s, has led to attempts to challenge the delegation of power to professional workers. Fuchs (1986) says that both government and corporate actors in health care in America have challenged the status quo on the basis that 'those who pay the piper should call the tune'. The capacity of funders, including government, effectively to constrain professional power, including its influence over technological innovation, may be affected by the structure of overall health care provision. The existence of controls within the public sector may have more impact upon the adoption and diffusion of technologies when the government is a major provider of health care services. Hollingsworth (1986) observes that despite the introduction of expensive technologies such as kidney dialysis and CAT scanners in Britain the use of these technologies has been quite constrained whilst both innovations have been used extensively in America. He argues that this difference is a reflection of public budgetary controls which exist in the two countries. The British health service budgetary system requires that innovations are carefully assessed against resource availability. In contrast the dispersed system of provision and funding in America makes attempts to exert controls over the direction of innovation and its related costs much more difficult to achieve.

Concern about the escalation of both private and public expenditure on health care in America since the 1960s has led to many attempts to exert greater control through federal action. In the early 1970s a system was introduced to allow professional monitoring of resource usage by individual physicians through the utilization review scheme. The National Health Planning and Resource Development Act 1974 sought to put in place a system for the collection and analysis of data on health needs. Related to this change was the requirement for states to examine proposals for expansion in hospital beds or identified capital investments in new technologies and to approve any changes by issuing a certificate of need (Bice, 1981; Hollingsworth, 1986). As the system of provision in Britain becomes more diverse, and the private sector contribution increases, it is interesting to see the debate emerge that new techniques for exerting government regulation over resource use within such an environment will have to be explored (Higgins, 1988).

Government mandating actions in relation to health care are most commonly found in a variety of health maintenance technologies in the workplace. Examples of these actions are the identification of physical building standards for factories and offices, the defining of safety standards for specific industries (requiring regular monitoring of the health of workers where hazardous work is involved) and in some instances the provision of direct health care services in the workplace. Provisions such as maximum working hours, annual holiday entitlement, sickness and accident payments, and maternity and paternity leave are all examples of actions which government may take to mandate the work environment. Employers are expected to respond to these mandates and to make various provisions often without any direct financial compensation from government. Outside the workplace government regulations also mandate the creation of private and public living space. Building and planning regulations determine what is acceptable in private and public arenas. Government also acts to prescribe behaviours which might threaten the health and life of individuals and communities such as the imposition of controls over those selling and consuming alcohol or tobacco products.

The identification of the health care goals which are to be mandated may not necessarily come from central government. The American Hospital Association's adoption and promotion of hospital insurance in the form of the Blue Cross programme required mandatory action from the states in order to provide the enabling legislation sanctioning the development of such programmes. Government action may also in effect mandate private providers where government itself plays no part in service provision. The adoption of Medicare made health insurance cover for the aged compulsory and it was funded by the federal government but the insurance policies as such were not provided by government. In effect private insurance operators were being mandated and fully reimbursed by the state for insuring a high risk section of the population.

The boundaries between government actions in mandating and supporting are sometimes difficult to identify. In Britain the 1911 National Health Insurance Act sought to achieve a balance between the interests of many groups - friendly societies, trade unions, insurance companies, health care professions and the government. The structure which was decided upon mandated an ongoing role for each party to play in the system of health care insurance for workers. One of the precursors of the legislation was the severe financial difficulty which many friendly societies were facing being caught between rising costs, increasing demand and inadequate income. Government action in effect supported those societies and ensured their continuance, at least for some time into the future. Another consequence of the legislation was to protect and increase the income of general practitioners which could be viewed as another example of support. The history of voluntary hospitals in Britain illustrates the links between support activity of government at both national and local level with periods of financial pressures on these institutions associated with major economic depressions in the 1870s/80s and 1920s/30s. Government responded by offering various forms of grants and subsidies to assist the hospitals. Governments have also played an important role in supporting research activities in medicine through direct funding in public institutions as well as supporting research and development by private sector research activities. Starr (1982, p. 348) has charted the dramatic rise of federal funding of medical research since the 1940s and these developments arc part of a much wider growth of federal funding of industrial research in America (Mansfield, 1977, p. 3).

The interaction of government and private sector provision has perhaps had greatest impact upon changing organizational and delivery technologies in health care through government stimulation of private provision by offering a variety of incentives. Private hospital and general medical insurance in America was predominantly in the hands of the Blue Cross and Blue Shield schemes during the 1930s and early 1940s. The federal government imposed a wage freeze during the Second World War but excluded fringe benefits from this restriction. It was during this period that dramatic growth occurred in employer contributions to group health insurance schemes. This trend was subsequently consolidated by trade union action which sought to make voluntary health insurance an important feature of collective bargaining in the postwar period. The fiscal treatment of employer contributions as a business expense and individual premiums as allowable against individual tax liability was, and remains, a major influence on the growth and operation of third party insurance in American health care.

The gradual growth of private sector health provision, including third-party insurance, has been an important facet of health care in Britain especially since 1965. Another feature of this growth has been the development of occupationally based health insurance schemes organized through employers or through associations of professional workers. The number of group schemes almost doubled from 403,000 to 793,000, during the period 1965–75 (Higgins, 1988, pp. 46–8). Many of the changes in the public/private mix in health care in Britain from the end of the 1970s have reflected the encouragement of change under a Conservative government. That encouragement has taken the tangible form of stimulating private health provision by the introduction of tax allowances for health insurance premium payments for companies. Similarly tax incentives to encourage the creation of small businesses have had an influence on health care service production. A growth in entrepreneurial activity in developing health care has also been stimulated in America. The system of administration of Medicare and Medicaid features a variety of tax allowances and exemptions, guaranteed returns on equity and reimbursements of interest on debt servicing (Hollingsworth, 1986, p. 74). The creation of health maintenance organizations also been encouraged through a mix of fiscal and other tangible forms of federal payments.

Linked to the mechanisms for stimulating private health care provision described above has been the parallel movement towards contracting and competitive tendering of social service provisions. These developments have grown strongly in America at both federal and state level since the beginning of the 1970s. The lack of a substantial role for direct service provision by federal or state authorities in health care places limits upon the scope that contracting from the public sector can play in the American health care system. In Britain contracting has occurred in health provision since the early 1970s. The potential role of contracting and tendering by government of various kinds of services ranging from ancillary support services to direct patient medical services is much greater because of the provider role of government which still accounts for about 90 per cent of all services. As with any innovation there are questions to be resolved including whether contracting should be stimulated or mandated by central government. The future potential contribution and the limitations of contracting and how these might affect the innovation and diffusion of organizational technologies in health care remains to be seen (Ascher, 1987).

GOVERNMENT AND CONVERGENCE OF HEALTH CARE SYSTEMS?

In earlier chapters the development of the technological base of modern health care has been briefly described. The diagnostic, treatment and maintenance technologies which have emerged since the nineteenth century have been widely adopted and diffused throughout industrially developed countries. The modern hospital, the operating theatre, diagnostic tests, drug treatments – these types of technologies are employed widely throughout those countries confirming that modern medicine is frequently based upon considerable uniformity in the adoption and diffusion of technologies. Historically, however, there have been major differences in organizational and delivery technologies in health care and governments have played an important role in each country in defining this aspect of technology. Governments act to define the organization of their own activities in the direct provision of health care, in the funding of health and in influencing the behaviour of other actors in health service provision.

Hollingsworth has observed that: 'The history of the British medical delivery system suggests that technology influences structure, for once there was a technology that was believed to be efficacious, the behaviour of private and public hospitals began to converge' (1986, p. 42). Hollingsworth is describing the way in which public hospitals in Britain during the 1920s and 1930s began to change. In the past these organizations had offered relatively poor standards of treatment because they were slow to adopt the technological innovations which were becoming available and which were being used in the voluntary hospitals. The acceptance of the potential of those technological innovations and their rather late adoption into public hospitals meant that the form and internal organization of all hospitals became more alike. Given the wider conception of technology which has been used in this analysis, this point again supports the proposition that innovations in part of the technological mix create opportunities for innovations elsewhere in the technological base which in turn may contribute to further changes. The availability of new technologies in diagnosis and treatment within hospital services led to changes in the public sector hospitals which organizationally had grown out of Poor Law institutions and traditions. These changes in the longer run made the major organizational innovation by the government of the National Health Service more viable because the differences between the hospitals being nationalized had been diminished as the technological base of the hospitals became more alike.

The health care systems in America and Britain and the role which government plays in these two systems appear to be quite disparate. Britain has followed the European development of social insurance and has emerged with universal coverage of the population for hospital and general medical care services and the government as the dominant provider of those services. America has looked to the individual consumer and private providers to meet health care needs and consumption has been backed by third-party insurers with employer and union involvement in this process.

The medical technologies that are employed by hospital and community health workers are dynamic and indeed seem constantly changing and improving. A question which has received considerable attention in recent decades is to what extent the patient's experience of health services reflects changes in the capacity of those services to modify his or her condition dramatically. It has already been noted that the 1960s and 1970s have seen a lively debate amongst critics and defenders of modern health care services as to the impact which many recent innovations have had upon health outcomes and the value of any modifications of health status relative to the costs of interventions. A rather different perspective on this debate is achieved by posing questions about the nature of changes in the technological base during recent decades. Has the technological base been transformed by a series of radical innovations in the same manner as the waves of innovations in the late nineteenth century and the 1930s and 1940s? Alternatively, are the innovations which have been adopted more accurately portrayed as mostly improvement innovations which are aimed at trying to realize the full potential of earlier changes? If the options for radical change in treatment, diagnostic and preventive technologies are not available at this time then improvement technologies combined with increasing emphasis and convergence on innovations in organizational technologies would not be unexpected. (The relationship between different types of health care innovation and cycles in economic activity will be discussed more fully in the next chapter.)

Government has a very important influence upon the organizational technologies used in social services such as health care. The questions faced by governments in looking at innovations may be different in different countries, but there are also similarities. How can access to health care be made available to all members of society, especially those who have limited financial means and those with special health needs? How can individual choice be given to consumers without losing social benefits or avoiding social costs associated with health care consumption which is below the social optimum? How can consumers be empowered relative to the position of providers given the imbalance of knowledge between the two? How can the costs of health care be controlled at a time when the demand on resources within national economies is high?

These are the kinds of questions which governments in Britain and America have confronted during the last twenty or thirty years. Medical science and other sources of innovation do not appear to have generated innovations which are perceived as allowing a transformation in the way that health care needs are met at this time. In these circumstances it is not surprising that the health care systems in America and Britain in recent years have become more alike rather than less alike as a result of government action. In other sectors of the economy increasing stagnation and similarity in the technological base between private sector producers of goods and services create the conditions for mergers and takeovers to occur. Faced with a similar situation in production of health care services attempts may be made to meld private and public sector provisions and in this process create greater organizational similarities between national health systems than existed prior to these conditions.

In America the federal government has been drawn into a more active role in health care in order to achieve greater access for a broad range of consumers through programmes such as

Medicare and Medicaid. These changes have led to a greatly increased funding role for federal government. The need to exert control over that expenditure has encouraged the initiation of a wide range of controls to be applied to providers. In Britain private health care insurance has grown dramatically and has been encouraged by government in both tangible and intangible ways. Alongside these changes in funding has been the emergence of increased private health provision. These provisions have included more private hospitals, rather than increasing the provision of private practice beds within national health hospitals and the entry of large American health care firms into both the health insurance and provision sectors of the British market. Health care services which had previously been provided publicly have been contracted out to private sector providers and opened up to competitive tendering. These are the organizational initiatives which are increasing private sector involvement in the British health system. These changes in the organization and delivery of health care in America and Britain do not mean that the two systems are identical or indeed ever likely to become so. The proposition is that they have become more alike than they were and that one reason for this is that given similar problems, and no fundamental alternatives in the rest of the technological mix, then the organizational technologies adopted will tend to become more alike.

5 Technological Change and Economic Cycles

INNOVATION AND ECONOMIC CYCLES

Economists have tried to identify and explain changes in economic activity which take place over time. Various theories putting forward the existence of trade and business cycles have emerged as a consequence of their endeavours. Rau (1974, p. 11) says that there are two major propositions about economic cycles about which there seems to be general agreement. The first is that expansions and contractions in the economy occur with major sectors moving up and down more or less together, and the second that these fluctuations have a discernible pattern and are not haphazard. A number of different cycles of varying lengths have been identified:

1 the Kitchen or inventory cycle with a length of 3–5 years
2 the Juglar or investment cycle with a length of 7–11 years
3 the Kuznets or building cycle with a length of 15–25 years
4 the Kondratieff or long-wave cycle with a length of 45–60 years

These cycles are named after those who first proposed their existence, which illustrates nicely the linkage between invention and inventor in public perceptions of invention. In general the shorter the time span of the cycle the greater the level of acceptance of its existence because the data necessary to validate the cycle exists, whilst verification of longer cycles, such as the Kondratieff, is much more problematic as only a relatively few cycles have occurred upon which to base an analysis.

Economic cycles, especially Kondratieffs or long waves, are important to an examination of technological innovation because of theories which claim that high rates of radical innovations may occur during economic depressions. The Kondratieff or long-wave cycle denotes a period of 45–60 years between major depressions in the world economy. Mensch (1979, p. 17) characterizes the downswing in economic activity with decreasing profit returns and lessening opportunities for improving the basic innovations of the past. He describes industrial development as 'a phase transition from one stalemate in technology to another with time spans of about two generations in between, during which diffusion and diversification of the new technologies run their course' (p. 17).

Mensch's analysis leads him to the view that basic innovations occur in swarms and that this swarming of innovations is most apparent during periods of economic depression (p. 131). The lack of basic innovations at other periods in the long-wave economic cycle is a reflection not merely of inadequacies in basic research and invention, but rather of the inadequacies of economic and political structures in disseminating information about available research and in committing capital to the realization of earlier inventions. The stagnation in products, processes and markets becomes apparent to all prior to a world economic crisis as capital and labour become under-utilized. It is only under this kind of demand-based pressure that basic innovations are actively sought and the conditions for capital commitment are achieved.

Mensch's analysis has been criticized on a number of counts (for example by Clark, Freeman and Soete, 1983; Delbeke, 1983; Rothwell and Zegveld, 1981). The data on which the analysis is based has been criticised as being inadequate and inaccurate. The ability to distinguish clearly between basic or radical innovations on the one hand and improvement innovations on the other has also been questioned. The heavy emphasis on demand pull as the cause of innovation is also criticized as being too near to being a mono-causal explanation.

Some alternative explanations, however, come close to pursuing single factor explanations as well. Clark and his colleagues

(1983, pp. 73–6) believe that the available evidence supports the importance of scientific discovery as the trigger for the swarming of innovations. A breakthrough in scientific discovery and technology may therefore be more closely related to periods of high consumer demand or war-induced expansion in consumption. Rostow (1983; van Duijn, 1983, pp. 83–92) places the major emphasis upon changes in the capacity to produce food and raw materials within the total world economy as the cause of long-wave activity. Other theorists focus upon the position of the factors of production during economic cycles, stressing the importance of either capital or labour. Forrester (1977; 1983) and the MIT System Dynamics Group place changes in the capital goods sector at the centre of their model. They argue that changes in capital investment in one sector of the economy will be transmitted through a multiplier effect to other sectors of the economy. Those who make capital investment decisions exaggerate this process by building up capital stocks rapidly in an economic upswing and collapsing investment and capital stocks in a downswing. Forrester believes that it is changes in capital stocks which occur over a period of about fifty years which are critical rather than changes in scientific knowledge or the rate of technological innovation. Mandel (1980; 1983), utilizing a Marxist framework of analysis, also emphasizes the role of capital accumulation, describing long waves as successive periods of accelerating and decelerating capital accumulation. During an upswing the rate and level of profit is increasing and the volume of capital increases until a point is reached where it is no longer possible to invest the total capital at an acceptable rate of profit, and underinvestment and economic depression occurs.

As has already been noted governments play an important role in the provision of capital for research and development. This funding assists in the identification of new knowledge, in examining its application and also in encouraging the realization of new technologies in production. Governments not only directly fund research and development work through universities, research institutes and government establishments but they also indirectly fund research and development work through direct payments and taxation incentives to industrial concerns. Mansfield (1977, p. 3) estimated that in 1974 about 40 per cent of research and development expenditure in private industry in America was financed through the federal government. He observed that where the output of an industry is linked to the defence of the state, including space exploration expenditures, then a much greater proportion of funding is provided by the state – approximately 80 per cent in 1973. A perceived threat to the state may also be an important element in the capital commitment process; as Kleinknacht states: 'The coincidence of innovation and war armament efforts with all its consequences is not accidental' (1983, p. 60). The central importance of the state in the provision of capital for welfare services and the role of such expenditures in responding to perceived internal threats to the state through social conflict are of obvious importance when considering innovation within the welfare state.

As van Duijn concludes: 'A complete explanation of the long wave has to rely on the interplay of innovation life cycles and infrastructural investment' (1983, p. 139). We have to explore how scientific and technical breakthroughs affect, and are affected by, the availability of capital and the level of demand for innovations when markets are saturated and available technologies have been fully developed. Even then the influence of labour as a factor of production has not been fully incorporated into such an analysis. Freeman, Clark and Soete (1982) have argued that labour factors are important and that they are related to the distinction between innovation in products and processes. They say that innovations which are backed by capital investment generate demand for particular forms of labour, labour which is often scarce. Total employment opportunities and wage levels are increased and over time there is pressure to substitute for labour and hence reduce labour costs. The effect of innovation on the demand for labour and cost of labour is clearly important when considering innovation in services which tend to be more labour-intensive than manufacturing. Freeman and his colleagues believe that the upswing period of the long wave is likely to be dominated by product innovations which generate employment opportunities. The downswing in contrast will see the domination of process innovations which improve quality and quantity of production whilst reducing costs, especially labour costs, through labour substitution. This linkage of product and process innovations to different phases in the long wave has been supported by the work of Kleinknecht (1983, p. 58).

A number of writers have stressed the importance of seeing major innovations as being interdependent. Forrester (1983, p. 131) argues that the bundle of technologies which are adopted in the upswing of the long wave will be highly integrated and mutually reinforcing, as with energy, transport and communication. Once the pattern of integration becomes established innovations which are not compatible with the emerging pattern are rejected and may not be realized until a subsequent upswing. Rogers (1983, p. 14) acknowledges that innovations may be closely related to one another in 'technology clusters'. Gershuny (1983a, pp. 55–9) agrees that innovations are clustered in groups and that the realization of these innovations collectively will depend upon the creation of the necessary infrastructure. This applies not just to the diffusion of a single innovation but also the realization of a cluster of innovations. The electricity supply system illustrates this point being important in its own right and as an infrastructure component for the realization of many of the innovations in domestic and entertainment services. Equally road and railway infrastructures were necessary for the realization of a range of innovations in private and public transportation.

HEALTH CARE INNOVATION AND LONG–WAVE CYCLES

Having described various economic theories concerning the relationship between technological innovation and long-wave cycles in economic activity we can now examine the relationship between innovations in the technological base of health care and these long-wave cycles. Long waves or Kondratieff cycles are obviously based on the proposition that a capitalist economic system will continually move from a period of prosperity, through to a period of major depression and back to prosperity. The duration of these cycles will vary from forty-five to sixty years although there may be some minor variation in the timing of the cycles between different countries. The examination and validation of long waves is problematic because of their duration and the fact that there are only a small number of 'cases' available for study. Interest in long-wave theories has been almost as cyclical as the waves themselves, with economic depressions proving the 'trigger' for renewed attention from various analysts. The formal literature on long waves has however made little apparent impact on the analysis of the development of welfare states in general, nor upon examining the production of specific social services such as health care. It is, however, worth noting that the social policy literature has alluded to a loose linkage between depressions and social reforms. The timing of the development of the early programmes and institutions of the welfare state in Europe towards the end of the nineteenth century, and of present welfare state structures in the 1930s and 1940s, has been related by commentators to the timing of major economic depressions.

This chapter explores the pattern of technological innovations in health care relative to periods of economic prosperity and depression. The discussion assumes the existence of Kondratieff or long-wave cycles. Readers who wish to take an 'agnostic', or indeed 'atheistic', position on the existence of such waves can adopt the less contentious assumption that there have been periods of both prosperity and major depressions in the world economy since the beginning of the nineteenth century. The timing of technological innovations within the welfare state relative to such points of depression or prosperity must be of interest, irrespective of whether these points are part of regular and recurrent cycles or not.

Before moving to discuss health care directly it is important to establish the timing of long waves since the late eighteenth century. Schumpeter was the first economist to pursue Kondratieff's ideas about long waves and much of the subsequent debate has been grounded in Schumpeter's work. Kuznets used Schumpeter's analysis to date the first three Kondratieff cycles and Table 5.1 is based on this analysis (Mensch, 1979, p. 39) and augmented by van Duijn's (1983, p. 155) dating of the beginning of the fourth cycle.

Table 5.1 Dating of Kondratieff or long-wave cycles

Kondratieff cycles	Prosperity	Recession	Depression	Revival	Growth factors
Industrial Revolution				
1787–1842	1787–1800	1801–13	1814–27	1828–42	Cotton Textiles Iron Steam Power
Bourgeois				
1842–97	1843–57	1858–69	1870–84/5	1886–97	Railways
Non-mercantilist				
1898–1947	1898–1911	1912–24/5	1924/5–39	1940–7	Electricity Automobiles
Fourth Kondratieff				
1948–	1948–65	1966–72	1973–		

The health industry, like other sectors of industrial economies, is involved in the production of goods and services,
indeed health care is a major component in the economies of
economically developed countries. Table 5.2 is derived from
the identification and dating of basic innovations in health care
which was described in Chapter 2. Innovations in diagnostic,
treatment and preventive areas represent product innovations in
the sense that a new theory or product is introduced into the
production of health care. Innovations in the organization and
delivery of health care are more akin to process innovations in
that the conditions under which services are provided is altered
by these innovations. The data in Table 5.2 essentially relates to
the final recovery phase of the first Kondratieff wave through
to the recession phase in the fourth Kondratieff. Table 5.3 links
the identified health innovations to their timing relative to long
wave phases.

What light, if any, does this analysis of the history of innovations in health care make to the debate about the relationship
between patterns of innovation and long waves in economic
activity? Economists who have attempted to include the health
industry in their analysis of long waves have confined their

Table 5.2 The timing of health care innovations

	Year
Diagnostic theories and techniques	
Stethoscope	1819
Microscope	1830
Haematology	1840–3
Ophthalmoscope	1850
Laryngoscope	1857
Cell Theory	1857
Medical thermometry	1860s
Immunology	1881
Bacteriology	1880s
X-rays	1895
Blood pressure measurement	1896
Blood group classification	1901
Electrocardiograph	1903
Electroencelphalograph	1929
Electron microscope	1933
DNA	1953
CAT scanner	1972
Treatment technologies	
Anaesthesia	1846
Aspirin	1853
Antisepsis	1867
Psychoanalysis	1900–10
Insulin	1920
Cortisone	1931
Anti-malaria drugs	1932
Sulpha drugs	1932
Penicillin	1940
Streptomycin	1943
Blood transfusion	1942–6
Psychotropic drugs	1952
Prevention and maintenance technologies	
Vaccination: Inoculation (smallpox)	1790s
Injection	1884
Diphtheria	1891
TB	1943
Rubella	1966
Water supply and waste disposal	1840s–50s
Fluoridation	1945
Contraceptive pill	1954
Rhesus haemolytic	1960

Table 5.2   *continued*

	Year
Organizational and delivery technologies	
General	
Acceptance of physical examination of the patient	1840s–50s
Specialization	1870s–90s
Training of nurses	1870s
Clinical laboratories	1880s
'Modern' hospital	Late 1870s–80s
Group practice	1890s
Neighbourhood health centres	1910–20
Computerization of patient records	1960s
Britain	
Formation of British Medical Association	1836
Public Health Act	1848
Friendly societies' direct employment of doctors	1870s
Introduction of pay beds in hospitals	Late 1880s–90s
National Health Insurance Act	1911
National Health Services Act	1946
British United Provident Association	1948
Tax relief on private health insurance premiums	1981
America	
Formation of American Medical Association	1846
Introduction of pay beds in hospitals	1880s
Food and Drug Act	1906
Blue Cross	1929
Blue Shield	Early 1930s
Government encouragement of employer/union third-party health insurance cover	Early 1940s
Medicare/Medicaid	1965
Health maintenance organizations	Late 1960s

The data in Table 5.2 essentially relates to the final recovery phase of the first Kondratieff wave through to the recession phase in the fourth Kondratieff. Table 5.3 links the identified health innovations to their timing relative to long wave phases.

attention predominantly, or exclusively, to pharmaceuticals and broader changes within the health industry have received minimal attention within this wider analysis. Van Duijn (1983, p. 187), for example, suggests that there is no evidence of a long cyclical pattern for 'medicines', but his comments are based solely on pharmaceuticals and include only a very small number of cases.

On the basis of Table 5.3 it does appear that there is a lower rate of innovation within health care during the recession phase of the long wave. The rate in the recession phase is less than the rate in all the other phases for each of the three

Table 5.3 Health care innovations and Kondratieff cycles

Kondratieff Cycles	Innovations excluding specific country innovations	Innovations with British structural innovations	Innovations with American structural innovations
2nd Kondratieff			
Prosperity 1843–57	6	7	7
Recession 1858–69	3	3	3
Depression 1870–85	8	9	9
Recovery 1886–97	4	5	5
3rd Kondratieff			
Prosperity 1898–1911	3	4	4
Recession 1912–24	2	2	2
Depression 1925–39	5	5	7
Recovery 1940–7	5	6	6
4th Kondratieff			
Prosperity 1948–65	5	6	6
Recession 1966–72	2	2	3

Kondratieff waves for which data is presented. The health industry does appear to follow the pattern apparent in the manufacturing sector of low levels of innovation as stagnation and recession affect national and international economic systems. The rate of innovation in the other three phases is less easily interpreted. There is a higher rate of innovation during the depression phase, but innovation appears to remain high during the recovery phase and to 'spill over' into the period of prosperity. The data offers support for both main theoretical explanations which stress technological innovation as critical in long-wave activity namely the depression-demand-generation model and the prosperity–pull argument.

Are the problems in interpretation a reflection of inadequacies of the data on innovation? There may be debate about what innovations should be included as representing important changes in the technological base of health care. Table 5.2 is based upon the general literature concerning the history of technology and the history of health care technology. Similar items have been included in other analyses of innovation. The inclusion of organizational and delivery technologies may be open to question concerning inclusions and exclusions. There could, however, be little argument about the importance of the 1911 and 1946 Acts in Britain or Blue Cross and Medicare and Medicaid in America. It is also important to recognize that the inclusion of these areas of change merely confirms the same pattern which exists if they were to be excluded from the analysis.

The dating of innovations does present difficulties and this is demonstrated by the variation in dating in the various sources that have been used. Despite this the variations are usually in the order of one or two years and would not fundamentally change the distribution of innovations. There are a few exceptions to this such as penicillin. Penicillin was discovered by Fleming in 1929 but it was not isolated and its potential medical uses realized until 1940 as a result of the work of Florey and Chain; very limited production began in 1941 (Hough, 1975, pp. 326–8). Large-scale production did not occur until 1944 in America when penicillin was used for treatment purposes during the Second World War. Some sources date the point of innovation as 1929 in the depression phase and others as 1940 in the recovery phase.

At this point it is appropriate to recall Usher's theory of 'cumulative synthesis' as an appropriate way to understand how knowledge is generated and applied. Knowledge building and application is a continuous process which may contain acts of insight which order that knowledge in new ways and represent a tangible break with the previous level of understanding. Given this view it is clear that whilst the division of technological change into the three phases of invention, innovation and diffusion may be a useful analytical tool, there are implicit difficulties in attempting to identify each phase with a specific point in time. They should be seen as representing overlapping and interacting elements in the total process of knowledge generation and application.

Another limitation of a single-industry analysis of innovation is that it concentrates on endogenous innovations and fails to recognize the effect of important exogenous innovations. This omission includes the clustering of innovations and infrastructure creation which may have a major impact on many areas of product and service production. The earlier description of the development of hospital- and community-based health care referred to various important exogenous innovations such as the development of rail and car transport and telephone communications systems. The influence of these innovations permeated the whole economic and social structure including the way in which health needs were met. The computer, since the early 1950s, has had a similarly pervasive impact in transforming the storage and analysis of information in all service industries including social services such as health. There may be a substantial time period necessary to establish the infrastructure necessary for the realization of these innovations, whose influence straddles many areas of activity. The impact of such innovations on a single industry like health care will be subject to time lags which will delay industry-specific innovations. These time lags may play a part in explaining the general shape of innovation in health care in which innovations are spread through the depression to prosperity phases of the long wave.

It is not possible to test the relative merits of explanations of the long wave based on changes in the pattern of capital availability, as opposed to variations in the demand or supply of technological innovations. The detailed breakdown of capital and current expenditures by private for-profit providers, voluntary and non-profit providers and public provision over the period of several long-wave cycles is not available. The behaviour of government in terms of the rate of growth in spending on health care provision and the allocation of that spending between capital and current expenditure might provide a partial test of the capital supply theory and a partial explanation for the high levels of innovation during the prosperity phase of the long wave.

GOVERNMENT ACTION, HEALTH CARE AND LONG WAVES

A number of propositions concerning government income and social spending in general, and health care in particular, during the long wave are outlined below. Some selective evidence is given in support of these propositions which, whilst not establishing their validity, does indicate that they warrant further more systematic research.

1   Government income will tend to rise more rapidly during the prosperity and recession phases of the long wave and government social expenditure will also tend to grow more quickly during these phases.

Government income is generated primarily from taxation levied upon the income and spending of individuals and companies. If, as is implied in both capital supply and innovation explanations of the long wave, the depression and recovery phases are when investment is made in innovations and improvement technologies then the emphasis at this time will be on investment and capital stock creation rather than generating current income and consumption. Such behaviour is more likely to be stimulated by government through various mechanisms which reduce taxation payments and encourage saving and investment and effectively reduce potential government tax income. Investments during the upswing in the long wave will be translated into enhanced personal and company incomes during the prosperity and early recession phases. As a result government income is likely to grow more quickly during the peak of the long wave covering parts of the recovery, prosperity and recession phases. As Freeman (1983) claims the demand for skilled labour is in general likely to be higher during the peak of the long wave. This effect may be particularly marked in social services such as health care where many innovations generate demands for skilled labour. Social expenditures, especially upon the labour component of social service provision, will tend to be relatively high at these times. Such a proposition is certainly supported by the earlier detailed discussion of the relative positions of capital and labour in health care innovation.

Evans (1983) cites the work of Mitchell and Deane on government income and expenditure data for England and Wales from 1781 to 1870. This data (Table 5.4) gives an indication of growth rates for government income and expenditure during the first long wave and the first two phases of the second long wave. Table 5.4 gives some credence to the notion that

Table 5.4 Government income and expenditure in England and Wales, 1781–1870

Time	Long-wave phase	Index of government income (1791–1800 = 100)	Index of government expenditure (1791–1800 = 100)
1781–90	Prosperity	73	57
1791–1800	Prosperity	100	100
1801–10	Recession	240	182
1811–20	Recession/ depression	318	227
1821–30	Depression/ recovery	266	152
1831–40	Recovery	236	145
1841–50	Prosperity	256	152
1851–60	Prosperity/ recession	292	181
1861–70	Recession	318	191

Source: Derived from Evans, 1983, p. 389.

both government revenue and expenditure will tend to expand most rapidly in the downswing of the long wave gathering a momentum which is sustained even into the first part of the depression.

Table 5.5 presents an index of the rate of growth of government revenues, total expenditure and social service expenditure relative to gross national product in Britain for the period from 1911 to 1975. This table provides a similar picture as that for the eighteenth and nineteenth centuries with the growth of government income and spending accelerating in importance in the total national economy during the prosperity and recession phases of the long wave and 'spilling over' into the initial part of the depression. The OECD (1985b, pp. 14–19) analysis of general income and expenditure trends from 1960 to 1981 in the seven major OECD countries confirms the pattern of acceleration in governments' income and to a greater extent spending, through the tail of the prosperity phase and into the recession and depression phases. The indications and expectations would then be that the rate of growth of income and spending on services such as health will be curbed as the depression phase becomes fully established (Fuchs, 1986, pp. 300–7). The annual

Table 5.5 Growth in government revenue, expenditure and social spending in Britain, 1911–75

Time	Long-wave phase	Index of government revenue	Index of government expenditure	Index of government social spending
		(indexes based on 1937 = 100)		
1911	Prosperity	46	49	39
1921	Recession	103	114	93
1931	Depression	105	112	117
1937	Depression	100	100	100
1951	Prosperity	179	175	148
1961	Prosperity	162	164	161
1971	Recession	204	196	218
1975	Depression	196	225	264

Source: Derived from Gough, 1979, table 5.1, p. 77.

growth rate of government social expenditures taking into account inflation has dropped from an average of 8.3 per cent during the period 1960 to 1975 to 4.3 per cent from 1975 to 1981 in the seven major industrial economies. The respective figures for Britain are 5.9 per cent to 1.8 per cent and for America 8.0 per cent to 3.2 per cent (OECD, 1985b, p. 21).

2   Political innovations in social services such as health care are more likely to occur during the end of the recovery phase, through the prosperity phase and the initial stages of the recessionary phase than at any other points in the long wave.

There are two main reasons for advancing this proposition. The first reason is the tendency for government income to build up during the end of the recovery and prosperity phases. The second reason is the increasing pressure for organizational changes which is stimulated by the various technological innovations which have occurred and are occurring during the depression, recovery and prosperity phases of the long wave. This transformation is seen as equivalent to that described by Freeman, Clark and Soete (1982) in which product innovations in the upswing of the long wave give way to process innovations which continue into the recession. In addition there are increasingly limited opportunities for further radical innovations and reducing returns from improvement innovations once the prosperity phase is reached.

If the first proposition is valid then it provides support for the second proposition. Governments have more money available to spend as the top of the long-wave cycle is achieved. In these circumstances government expenditure, including social expenditure, will frequently continue to accelerate during the early recessionary phase and indeed into the initial years of the depression. This indicates that governments are most likely to see themselves as being in a position to fund changes in their social service activities at this time and the expenditure implications of these decisions will then flow on through the recession and into the beginning of the depression.

Public demands for government to extend the coverage of social services and to improve the quality of services is likely to build up during the depression and recovery phases of the long wave. The incidence of illness, especially in low-income households, is likely to have increased during the depression (Richardson, 1945) as will have general mortality, morbidity and the incidence of psychiatric illnesses (Liem, 1981). Consumer demand may also increase as a variety of technological innovations become available through the depression and recovery phases. Fuchs and Kramer (1972, p. 14) argue that there is a latent demand for health which becomes transformed into market demand when appropriate technologies are generated. Pressure may come not just from service users. Providers, such as hospitals and doctors, find their incomes under pressure during the depression periods and faced with this situation they are likely to seek ways of maintaining consumption and protecting their future income levels (Richardson, 1945). As well as modifying their own behaviour providers may lobby government to intervene in the market.

The momentum of demand and lobbying pressures upon government are likely to take time before they elicit action unless there is wide agreement about the necessity and form which intervention should take (Polsky, 1984). Rothwell and Zegveld (1981, p. 17) argue that depressions often stimulate a structural crisis in the various sectors of an economy and such structural problems have frequently been associated with a transformation in the role of government. This kind of transformation has been apparent in health care even though there is clearly a substantial time lag between the depression and changes in government actions and institutions.

Political innovations either lay down the rules under which providers of services, including government itself, will operate or they influence and create the organizational structure for that activity. Even though product innovations may 'swarm' during the depression or the recovery–prosperity phases of the long wave there are further reasons for expecting political innovations to come towards the end of this sequence. Political innovations which modify the organizational environment can be viewed as responses to the opportunities created or the changes made necessary by the flow of technical and non-technical innovations. Innovations in an industry such as health care can change the types of services and products available, the form in which they are available and the cost of providing the service. Major political innovations in health care are part of organizational innovations which modify the market by changing consumer access to health care and extending coverage within the national population as well as the conditions under which producers operate. The extension of coverage is an important component in the commitment of social expenditure; for example 4.1 per cent of the 10.3 per cent annual growth rate of health care spending in America from 1960 to 1975 is attributable to extension of coverage and this has been

Table 5.6 Major political innovations in British and American health care systems

	Innovation	Year	Long-Wave Phase
Britain	Public Health Act	1848	Prosperity
	National Health Insurance Act	1911	Prosperity/recession
	National Health Services Act	1946	Recovery (implementation prosperity)
	Federal encouragement of third-party health insurance through tax relief	1940s	Recovery/ prosperity
America	Medicare/Medicaid	1965	Prosperity/recession

particularly marked after the introduction of Medicare and Medicaid (OECD, 1985a, p. 40). Whilst organizational and political innovations are likely to be responsive to other types of innovations it must be remembered that they in turn may help stimulate future non-organizational innovations in the next long wave.

Table 5.6 can hardly be taken as conclusive proof of the proposition about the timing of government innovations. However, the major actions of government in the two countries which have changed the level of access to health care and the contribution of government either through direct provision or funding of other providers have occurred around the peak of the long wave either on the turning point between recovery and prosperity, during prosperity or on the turn between prosperity and recession. This association between government innovation and the long wave warrants further examination across a wider range of social expenditures.

3. Capital expenditure on health care in general and government expenditure in particular are more likely to occur during the upswing (depression → prosperity) of the long wave rather than the downswing (prosperity → depression).

The lack of detailed data on the division of expenditure between capital and current components over time makes it only possible to comment superficially on this proposition. Hospital construction, which is the major capital commitment component in health care, appears to have been concentrated in the mid-depression to mid-prosperity in both the third and fourth Kondratieff waves and this would be so in both America and Britain. Wohl's (1983, p. 162) figures for loans sanctioned by the Local Government Board for public health purposes between 1871 and 1897 which involved predominantly capital works provides some support for the proposition. The annual rate of growth in these loans during the depression phase of 1871–85 was 64 per cent whilst the growth rate dropped to just less than 13 per cent for the recovery phase of 1886–97. The balance between expenditure on capital and expenditure on labour in health care is an area where research would be of great value. There are still questions such as how does the balance change in relation to economic cycles including the long wave? Does a move towards spending relatively more on labour reflect a search for the full realization of all existing technologies in the face of a decreasing rate of basic innovations? Answers to these, and other questions, would greatly improve our understanding of innovation in health care and the relationship of innovation in health care to changes in the total economic structure.

It is important to restate that the exploration of technological change in health care and the relationship between innovation and long-wave economic cycles is not meant to imply that the evolution of health care is purely a reflection of these influences. There are numerous other variables at work and many of these have received careful analysis. One of those influences is the impact of warfare and this factor is important to an analysis of technological change in health care because of the possibility of a linkage between war and technological change. Mensch (1979, pp. 74–83) incorporates the notion that wars may be a 'signal' of a pending world economic recession in his theory of swarming of innovations during a depression. Wars have generated economic problems in countries in the immediate postwar period as they try to adjust from a wartime to a peacetime environment. In order to support his position Mensch cites the so-called 'reconversion crisis' in those countries which had defeated Napoleon in 1815, the *crédit mobilier* crisis in 1866 in the aftermath of the Crimean and European wars from 1854 to 1866, in America the repercussions of the Civil War from 1864 to 1866, the economic problems in the 1920s of those countries involved in the First World War, and finally the repercussions of the Vietnam War upon the American economy in the early 1970s. Mensch acknowledges that the Second World War does not fit this general model of wars occurring during the stagnation associated with the recession phase of the long wave and a subsequent signal economic crisis foreshadowing an imminent depression.

Other analysts have noted the importance of warfare in the pattern of technological change. Kleinknecht (1983) uses Mahdavi's identification of innovations as the basis of his analysis and Mahdavi identifies those innovations which received substantial support from government. Kleinknecht notes that in all cases an important catalyst to government support was the wish to respond to war conditions or the threat of impending warfare.

There can be no doubt that wars have influenced innovations in health. Nursing practice and the need for training was affected by nursing experience during the Crimean War. In America, hospital building programmes and conditions within the hospital were influenced by the Civil War. In Britain, the evidence of poor levels of health amongst substantial sections of the population was highlighted during the Boer War and, with the perceived threat of future war in Europe, was one of the factors leading to the introduction of national health insurance in 1911. The Second World War in particular affected the adoption and diffusion of technologies as well as stimulating experimentation and new technologies across a broad range of health care activities from new drugs such as penicillin to surgical techniques like blood transfusion and wider developments in psychiatry and psychological medicine.

PART II

Technology and the Welfare State

6 Technology and the Welfare State: A Missing Dimension

EXPLANATIONS FOR THE WELFARE STATE

Almost twenty years ago Robert Pinker (1971) highlighted the lack of any substantial theoretical underpinning to the various accounts for the historical development of welfare states and in the analysis of social policy questions. He described the way in which the history of the study of welfare institutions and policies had been based on empirical research and pragmatism in order to combat what were seen as the undesirable effects of social theory, and especially the social and economic implications of laissez-faire market theories (Pinker, 1971, p.50).

In the absence of any major concern about theory a simple evolutionary perspective on the welfare state tended to pervade both academic and public policy circles. The welfare state has been represented as a necessary and inevitable institutional consequence of industrialization in this evolutionary perspective. It has also been viewed as reflecting more enlightened social attitudes in which mutual obligations within the community have been increasingly recognized. Although there may be evidence of past deficiencies in the realization of social policies, an evolutionary perspective leads to a belief that these difficulties can be overcome in time through changing social attitudes and improved policy implementation. The welfare state has been a critical component in the evolution of a more enlightened society in which a set of social goals has been pursued which has had overwhelming public support. The limitations of this simplistic view have been highlighted by many other writers as well as Pinker (for example, Baker, 1979; Carrier and Kendall, 1973; Townsend, 1976). There has been increasing recognition of the need for greater attention to be paid to establishing a theoretical framework for studying the welfare state and social policy development.

There can be little argument that substantial progress has been made during the last twenty years in constructing theoretical accounts for why welfare states have appeared in economically developed countries. This progress has been apparent in a burgeoning literature offering historical and contemporary analysis and encompassing comparative as well as single-country accounts. It is not appropriate to review this literature in any detail here, since a wide range of explanatory factors have been used to illuminate the reasons for similarities and differences between national welfare states. Theoretical accounts have also encouraged a more critical approach to evaluating the aims and achievements of modern welfare states since their inception around the middle of this century. For example, Marxist theorists have turned their attention to the role of welfare in capitalist societies and questioned the claimed distributional impact of welfare provisions for the least well off, and the effectiveness of the 'social wage' for the working class in general. Ironically the interest in theory during this period has seen the re-emergence of the very 'normative theory of political economy' against which Pinker says the social reformers of the nineteenth and early twentieth centuries fought. This renaissance carries with it clear criticisms of the present scope of government action in the economy and society in general and specific criticisms of the provisions and controls imposed through the welfare state.

Technology and technological change have not featured prominently as a focus for direct attention in the range of explanatory models for the welfare state which have emerged. Where technology is included in the explanatory framework the analysis is limited and seems to reflect remnants of the simplistic evolutionary perspective described above. Our explanations for the welfare state appear generally to accept what Hindess (1987) refers to as the centrality or 'essentialism' of the market and with it the assumed links between economic growth and economic development. Consideration of the impact of technology has been largely confined to the indirect role which it is thought to have played in the process of industrialization. Industrialization in turn has been seen as generating changes in social and political institutions alongside the impacts of urbanization and related demographic changes. Descriptions of the effects of technological change have been broadly similar irrespective of whether the account is based on general theories of industrial society or capitalist society, although the explanations as to why such changes have occurred differ widely (Giddens, 1982). Invention and technological innovation are assumed to have been important in stimulating industrialization and in the generation of economic growth. The primary focus of analysis, however, has been on the role of economic growth in providing the conditions for continuing expansion in the industrial base and in generating an ongoing increase in resources which can be used to achieve the redistributive objectives of welfare state policies.

Many political changes have occurred alongside industrial-ization, including changes in the structure and operation of party politics and in the institutions of government. These changes have had important implications for the development of welfare state policies and institutions (see Ashford, 1986; Browning, 1986, for example). The focus here, however, is on the effect of economic change rather than political change. The need of industrial enterprises for predictability in their economic environment has been seen as contributing to the growth in government at both central and local level. Since the nineteenth century, government interventions in the economy have become increasingly extensive and have included measures to influence the operation of the labour market. Governments have acted to provide and regulate the provision of social services such as health, education and housing. Social security schemes have also been widely adopted which provide a degree of income security to citizens experiencing a variety of contingencies such as industrial accident, sickness, disability and unemployment. These schemes together with other social service provisions form the basis of the welfare state which is such a prominent feature in the institutional landscape of economically developed countries (Wilensky, 1975).

Most accounts for the welfare state treat technology and technological change as essentially exogenous variables which only affect the welfare state indirectly through their impact on economic growth, the process of industrialization and the kind of related social and political changes described above. These explanations place the welfare state at the end of a chain of events which are presented schematically in Figure 6.1.

This schema describes a basis for the continued evolution and development of an industrial and post-industrial society which is driven by technological change and consequent economic growth. The welfare state is portrayed in this schema as one of a series of social and institutional changes which are determined by the needs of the industrial system. Technology is therefore being viewed as a relatively minor component in an essentially hierarchical and deterministic model of an evolving industrial society. Technological change, however, is being ascribed a role in accounting for the development of welfare states, although this influence is confined entirely to that of an exogenous variable. Technology is the driving force behind industrial development and governments respond to the requirements and consequences of industrial development. The emergence and development of the welfare state is merely one of those governmental responses. There may be differences in the mechanisms used to deliver services in welfare states in different countries, but the circumstances under which help is given are thought to become more and more alike.

De Swaan (1988) notes that by the late 1930s the major options for organizing and funding welfare state activities had

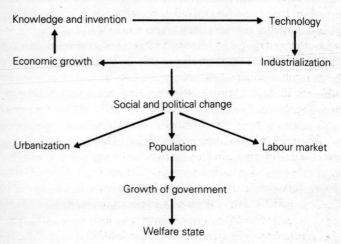

Figure 6.1   Welfare as a product of economic and technical change.

been experimented with by all Western governments. Welfare state activities are one of many ways in which industrial societies could be seen to converge (Mishra, 1977, pp. 33–43). The role of technology is that of an external 'given' whose impact on welfare is mediated through a variety of social and political institutions. Whilst these views are most evident in functionalist or convergence theories of the welfare state many of the assumptions concerning technological change, economic growth and industrial development appear in other theoretical accounts, including those of many Marxist commentators.

There are many examples of writers who have sought to establish a more complex relationship between technological change in industrial and economic systems on the one hand and social change, including aspects of the welfare state, on the other. Titmuss, (1974; 1976), for example, described the important growth of what he termed 'created' or 'man-made' dependencies which can stem from the realization of scientific technological changes. Unemployment, accidental injury and compulsory retirement are examples of the costs, or 'diswelfares' as Titmuss terms them, which may arise from the application of technological changes to industrial production. These contingencies may increase dependency for individuals and family groups and create pressure for government action. Social services can be seen as representing attempts to compensate people for the personal costs or diswelfares which have been generated through changes in the industrial system. Ester Boserup (1981), in her study of technological change and population, acknowledges that invention and technology have had important effects upon the size and distribution of population. However, she also argues that the size and structure of populations have historically been important factors in influencing the rate of technological innovation itself, and the speed and extensiveness of diffusion of those innovations. She offers an extensive analysis to support her position including discussion of agriculture, manufacturing, transport and health care. Kenneth Boulding (1981) has highlighted a complex relationship between the development of new technologies and changes in social institutions. He says: 'The development of new technologies and commodities likewise produced changes in organization and social structure, which in turn reacted on the new technologies' (p. 143).

The role of technological innovation described by these and other writers opens up the possibility of several feedback mechanisms operating within the schema identified in Figure 6.1. Changes within the industrial–economic system may stimulate changes in social and political institutions which subsequently affect the form and speed of technological innovation in industry. Whilst this modification recognizes the interaction between changes in social and political institutions, such as the welfare state and the industrial complex, the analysis still remains grounded in an essentially hierarchical perspective. Technological innovation continues to be perceived as an event which is completely exogenous to an institution such as the welfare state. Innovation may have indirectly affected the growth of the modern welfare state, and the existence of feedback mechanisms opens up the possibility that changes in the welfare state may in turn have influenced the process of technological innovation within industry. This kind of analysis remains severely limited because it ignores the role of the welfare system in the production of goods and services within the economy, and the fact that this production is based on a particular set of technologies at any point in time. It equally fails to recognize the role of social innovation, including organizational change, as a form of technological change rather than as a consequence of other types of innovation.

This lack of adequate recognition of the role which technology plays in the production of goods and services within the welfare state is a serious deficiency in our understanding of the history of the welfare state and its present operation. It can be argued that welfare state activities differ from other kinds of production in several ways. Some services and goods may have the characteristics of public goods or merit goods where questions about the social benefits of consumption or the social costs of not consuming are viewed as a justification for these goods to be publicly provided. The traditional activities of welfare in terms of education, health, housing, income support and personal counselling and support services can be seen as special because they seek to ensure that the basic needs and well-being of members of society are ensured. The term welfare state implies government involvement and government, whether at central, local, state or regional level may be the dominant provider or funder of the service. Consumption of social services may be at zero cost to users at the point of consumption or the cost may be modified by a wide variety of interventions by government.

Irrespective of these and other ways in which goods and services produced within the welfare state can be distinguished from those which are produced elsewhere in the economy, the central fact remains that goods and services are being produced. What is produced in the welfare system and the way in which it is produced relies upon a technology and that technology will change over time. Producers of social services such as health care have to address similar questions to other producers as to the range of products, services and production processes which are going to be utilized. Even if government were a monopoly producer of social services it would, like private sector monopolists, have to pay attention to the protection and development of its production technology. As has been demonstrated in health care the producer structure is far from being a monopoly situation with a complex pattern of public, private and non-profit producers, marketed and non-marketed services and products, and many intermediate goods and services being produced. This picture is similar to that which occurs in many other areas of social service production. The level of consumption of social services may be affected by government actions which modify the cost to consumers. Social services are not unique in this respect, however, as government interventions in the form of import tariffs, quotas, export incentive payments, tax allowances and so on have an impact on a wide range of goods and services. Government modification of the availability and cost of goods and services to consumers is not a reason for failing to study the technological base of an industry. Social service production in general, and the health care industry in particular, is of considerable importance within the economies of developed countries. These services are important employers of labour and other resources.

One of the ways in which an understanding of the development of particular industries and groups of industries has been enhanced is through examining the role of technological change and the relationship between technological change and broader changes in the overall functioning of national economies. A similar analysis of the technological base and changes in that technology over time for all the major activities within the welfare state has a part to play in increasing our knowledge of how the welfare state has developed and currently operates. A study of innovation in the welfare state should also take account of the possible relationship between changes in economic activity which are evident in long wave cycles in the economy and the rate of technological innovation in social service production.

The search for scientific knowledge and technologies generated by that knowledge is intrinsic to the notions of progress and enlightenment which have dominated social values in industrialized countries during the nineteenth and twentieth centuries. The foundations of individual social services such as health care and the total welfare state complex have been strongly influenced by this conception of progress. David Roberts (1960, p. 103), for example, has emphasized two elements as being crucial to the growth of public welfare institutions in nineteenth century Britain: first, advances in scientific knowledge, and second the belief in the possibility of human progress in general, and social progress in particular. Science and technology have been seen as the key which will unlock the door to human betterment as new goods and services and methods of production open up the prospect of freedom from material want. Just as the physical world could be understood and potentially harnessed to human objectives so too the social world might be susceptible to similar analysis and control through application of both the physical and social sciences.

The history of health care during the last 200 years clearly demonstrates the influence which science and technology have exerted upon our understanding of health and illness, for instance in the use of machine analogies to understand the operation of body organs. Our perception of appropriate health care has mirrored the increasing dominance of 'scientific medicine' amongst health care professions, the health industry and the community in general. The values upon which welfare states are grounded may stress social obligations between citizens but they also rest upon the assumption that collective action has, and will increasingly offer, the capability of alleviating and resolving human problems and enhancing individual and social well-being. The welfare state is a vehicle for collective action and government has a particular role in identifying the goals of well-being and then producing the technical solutions to achieve these goals. The linkages between the growth of welfare states, our conception of social progress and betterment and the role of science and technology are closely intertwined and an analysis of the welfare state should take account of these relationships.

No attempt has been made in this book to claim that changes in the welfare state can be attributed solely to technological change and the interaction between technological change, economic change and the welfare complex. What is asserted is that the present handling of technological change in accounts of welfare state developments is totally inadequate. These accounts offer no conceptualization of technology and technological innovation, whilst assuming that technological change in the economy has had a crucial impact upon the evolution of the welfare state. Whatever the orientation of accounts for the welfare state – the centrality of political structure, political process, class interest and so on – the acceptance of a simplistic and deterministic view of technology is a serious limitation in these accounts. This book has explored the process of technological innovation in health care and this analysis has revealed insights which can be incorporated into a wider account of welfare state development. As will be seen, these insights can also contribute to the contemporary debate concerning the 'crisis' of the welfare state.

TECHNOLOGY AND HEALTH CARE: AN OVERVIEW

At this point it may be helpful to summarize briefly the main points which emerged from the analysis of the effect of technological change on the development of health care services in Britain and America in Part I of this book.

Invention, innovation and diffusion of health care technology

Technology was defined as the various ways in which it is possible to replace, enhance or facilitate human functioning. The generation of new knowledge, and the application of that knowledge to the production of goods and services, was described as a process of 'cumulative synthesis'. Knowledge is built up over time with occasional discontinuities when new insights change our understanding of that knowledge. Invention is not an inventory of the discoveries of famous people but a process in which the insights and discoveries of those people advance the continuing process of knowledge building. Similarly the application of knowledge to production through innovation involves both the ongoing generation of solutions to perceived problems and innovations which introduce new ways of constructing and responding to problems.

The literature on technological innovation divides the process into three phases;

- invention in which new knowledge is generated
- innovation in which that knowledge is applied to the production of goods and services
- diffusion in which the new technology spreads through a system of potential users

This framework has been used to explore technological change in health care services whilst acknowledging the inherent limitations of segregating an ongoing process, in which complex feedback mechanisms operate, into discrete parts. Those innovations which represent a substantial change from existing products and production processes and which lead to new production activity have been termed radical or basic innovations. Other innovations represent improvements in existing technologies and they improve the quality or quantity of the goods or services which can be produced.

Health care technology was classified into four areas:

- diagnostic technologies
- treatment technologies
- maintenance and preventive technologies
- organizational and delivery technologies

The final category of organizational innovation is often overlooked but it is important because technological innovation cannot be understood without both recognizing the social context within which innovation occurs and the innovations in the social environment itself. Organizational innovations include changes in the way goods and services are marketed and managed as well as innovations in government policies. Changes in government policy and administration are of considerable significance in health care production. There are reasons to believe that organizational innovations may have increasing significance in the total process of innovation as industrial development proceeds (Boserup, 1981, p. 210).

Major changes in health care technology were identified and as far as possible their points of invention and innovation dated. The notion of a flow of improvement innovations following an initial basic innovation is easily illustrated in health care, for example in the development of antibiotic and psychotropic drugs or in diagnostic tools such as the stethoscope. It was observed that clustering of basic innovations can occur once the required infrastructure for the achievement of these innovations is in place. These groupings of innovations can exert immense influence upon technologies across many areas of economic activity. Historically, innovations in communication and transportation have had a pervasive effect throughout national economies and their influence has certainly been apparent in changes in health care.

Studies of the diffusion of innovations in manufacturing industries have emphasized such issues as the availability of capital and the rate of return generated by investment in an innovation. These factors are important in health care innovations but they are modified by the presence of non-profit producers such as church and voluntary organizations as well as public providers which means that not all providers will solely be seeking to maximize their rate of return. Another factor in assessing profit and capital commitment requirements in health care innovation is the role which government plays in modifying market conditions, for example through direct and indirect funding of research and development. These kinds of interventions affect both the cost of innovation as well as the likely rate of return on an investment. The diffusion of innovations in health care technology has been influenced by possible changes in the level of demand which has been a reflection not only of changes in population and per capita income but also in organizational innovations by private and

public providers. These providers have from time to time
increased their coverage of the population through modifying
the level and method of consumer payment. Diffusion, and the
speed with which diffusion takes place, has often been linked
to the quality of the labour force. Health care is dominated
by professional and technical workers who have high levels
of formal education. These workers usually prize continuing
training, their occupational cultures stress information sharing
and they have mechanisms to effect this information sharing
which have been established over a long period of time.

The way in which innovations in health care are adopted
and diffused was illustrated by describing three broad areas of
innovation since the mid-nineteenth century, first the development of the modern hospital, second, some changes in general
community-based medical practice and third, selected aspects
of non-product innovations in the pharmaceutical industry. The
description of innovation in both America and Britain helped
to highlight similarities and differences in the way innovations have occurred in two quite different health care systems.

Production, consumption and health care technology

The locus of production   Technological change removed health
care production from within the confines of the domestic household and transferred it into large, specially designed centres of
production just as had occurred in the production of other goods
and services during industrialization. Health care production
for much of the nineteenth century was home-based and the
experience of health care services was related to social class.
The wealthy could use domestic servants to provide physical care and purchase the services of a doctor to attend the
patient at home. The patronage of the wealthy was important to individual doctors if they were to achieve a reasonable level of income and therefore the patient retained some
measure of power and influence over the relationship between
doctor and patient. For the majority of the population, however, access to medical knowledge was acquired by referring
to popular medical publications and through the experience of
family members or local people who would provide services for
little or no payment. Control over the production of health

care rested within the household. Only the poorest members of society were cared for outside the household within the health care institutions of the Poor Law.

The complex web of innovations which became available during the nineteenth century enabled the locus of health care production to be gradually transferred from the household and into the hospital and general practice during the latter part of the nineteenth and early twentieth centuries. With the transfer of production went the transfer of power as control within hospitals was successively exercised by lay committees of subscribers, doctors, medical administrators and government officials. This control was symbolically represented by the careful regulation of contact between the patient and members of his or her family. The links between innovation in health care technology and the transfer of the location and control over production from the household to the health institution are well illustrated by the changes in childbirthing practices which have taken place since the middle of the nineteenth century.

Capital commitment and technological innovation The formalization of health care production outside the household has required the generation of capital to construct and equip hospitals and general practices. Developments across the whole spectrum of medical technologies have required capital commitment. Examples of innovations which have commanded substantial capital injection have included innovations in the development and manufacture of pharmaceuticals, the production and purchase of machinery required for diagnostic and surgical interventions and factory modifications to protect occupational health.

Producer assessments of the risk and profitability of these new technologies are influenced by the particular characteristics of the health care market. The availability of capital is not merely a function of the financial position of the producer or the ability of the producer to borrow. Philanthropic giving by the wealthy and from interest groups based upon particular medical conditions or local community interest have provided funds based upon factors other than risk and profit. The reputation of non-profit organizations for innovative action may also have played a part in decisions as to whether to pursue an innovation or not. The health care market is a complex one in which there are many producers of direct and intermediate goods and services. The reactions of the various 'players' must be assessed by potential innovators; for example, the reaction of health insurers and mutual benefit groups to an innovation are important as these intermediate institutions influence the funding of consumpption.

Government plays a particular role in determining the rules under which the health care market operates. It also has a more direct impact through the various ways in which it affects the availability and cost of funding and therefore the cost of developing and realizing innovations. Where government is a direct service provider and is faced with the capital commitment decisions of a producer, the political process of public policy decision making is likely to entail factors other than those which exist outside the public arena.

Labour influences upon technological innovation Labour as the other factor of production will also affect the decision to pursue and adopt an innovation and the speed of diffusion amongst producers. The quantity and quality of labour will affect the propensity to innovate. Health care has become an increasingly important employer of labour during the twentieth century both in direct employment and indirectly through the pharmaceutical industry and the production of intermediate goods and services for use in the health industry. The numbers employed in the major occupational groups have grown in absolute terms during this period but this masks important differences within these occupations. Since 1910, nursing and subsequently technicians have been the numerically dominant groups in the American health care labour force. These changes partially reflect first the transfer of the locus of production from the household and the provision of caring services within the hospital, and second the increasing importance of machines in direct and indirect patient care.

There are various reasons why labour is likely to be receptive to and indeed demand innovation. Health care occupations, to varying degrees, have formal entry requirements in which minimum educational levels are required. Science has been accepted as the appropriate framework within which to define and pursue knowledge and medical knowledge is claimed to be based upon scientific research. The pursuit of knowledge requires specialization amongst researchers and practitioners. Demonstrating knowledge and contributing to furthering that knowledge represent important ways in which the status of health care occupations are promoted and within occupations the status of individual practitioners established. If promotion and individual status are acquired in this manner then innovations which highlight the contribution of individual workers and affect 'cures' for individual patients with acute conditions are likely to be prized.

The substantial period of formal education required for initial entry to health professions and the ongoing expectation of continuing education epitomize the high levels of resources committed to promoting the quality of the health care workforce as well as its quantity. The quality of the workforce affects the capacity of an industry to adopt new technologies. In general the higher the quality of labour then the lower the costs of innovation in terms of the ability of the workforce to learn the new technology. Professional values which stress the search for knowledge and the sharing of that knowledge amongst the professional community will also facilitate innovation and diffusion of technologies. High geographical mobility, which also tends to occur in professional occupations, hastens the transmission of knowledge across national and international boundaries. The segregation of the labour market between occupational groups and within occupations by specialties may, however, partly offset the propensity to innovate. Labour may be geographically mobile but there will be little movement across inter- and intra-occupational boundaries which are jealously guarded by workers. These boundaries will tend to slow down the adoption and diffusion of innovations.

Research indicates that health workers are generally proactive towards the adoption and diffusion of innovations. Innovations in diagnostic and treatment technologies for those with acute conditions seem most likely to be encouraged whilst there may be resistance to organizational technologies which threaten established boundaries within and between occupations. In general innovations in health care appear to have generated complementary demands for labour rather than creating capital which substitutes for labour. This is apparent both in the growth of technical employment in health care and the creation of technical specialties within the established health care professions. To what extent this situation might reflect the limitations of existing health care technology rather than the relative positions of capital and labour in the industry can be debated.

An influence upon the current and future demand for labour in the formal health services is the ageing of the population and alongside this increasing numbers of the working population in late middle age who will experience chronic conditions which require long-term medical and nursing care. The availability of labour through the informal system within the household has been affected by changes which have occurred within the household in industrial countries. These changes include the smaller size of households, the incidence of divorce and remarriage, and the increase in sole-parent households. In addition changes in female participation rates in the formal workforce have had major implications for the availability of informal care within the household. In the absence of labour-substituting technologies these changes have important implications for the health care industry and other areas of social service provision.

Consumption and technological innovation   The perception of what health needs exist and how these needs can be met have varied between different sections of society. From the point of view of producers, whether individual doctors, groups of community-based practitioners, hospitals or drug companies, their existence relies upon the consumption of their services and being paid a sufficient rate to generate an acceptable income. The history of the development of hospital and general practice in both Britain and America shows that service producers have never lost sight of this requirement and the need to look for marketing and management innovations. In the nineteenth century hospitals in Britain sought to develop special funds through payments from workers and church congregations to supplement their subscription income from wealthy patrons. Faced with financial problems during the economic depression of the 1920s American hospitals acted individually and collectively to enable more Americans to have access to hospital care in a manner they could afford through the creation of

Blue Cross. These and other innovations, especially in social insurance and third-party coverage of health care, demonstrate the importance of innovations in the organization and delivery of services. These innovations have frequently modified the ability of consumers to use services through marketing and managerial changes.

Future innovations may transform the consumption of health services. Some writers believe that the traditional methods of health care production may change in the foreseeable future. Current technology relies upon hospital provision with face-to-face service involving high levels of labour for both direct and indirect services. Innovations in interactive communication technologies and computer software capabilities may incorporate elements of a new infrastructure which will allow consumption of health care to be partly returned to the domestic household despite the changes that have taken place and are taking place in family life.

Government policy and innovation

All changes in government policy which affect health care represent forms of innovation in the organization and delivery of the service. The evolution of the welfare state is part of the wider growth in the scope of government intervention in many aspects of everyday life. Just as with other forms of technological change, innovations may be of a minor nature in which small changes are made with the objective of improving existing systems, or the changes may represent a more fundamental change in the way in which services are organized.

The role of governments in the health care systems of America and Britain seem to be quite different. The British system is based upon the concept of social insurance and involves direct government activity in service provision as well as action to fund access to health care. The 1911 and 1946 Acts represented major political innovations in which government moved to increase access to health care culminating in free, universal access. Government involvement in providing health services was increased and government established as the central organizing and management agency. The American health system and the role of the federal government appears quite different from the British experience. The federal government has no major role in service provision and state and local bodies are only minor producers amongst a complex structure of for-profit and non-profit providers. The concept of social insurance has not been accepted despite attempts to introduce it by different groups several times during the twentieth century. The introduction of Medicare and Medicaid in 1965, however, did represent a major innovation with government funding access to health care for a substantial section of the American community.

Governments influence health care services in less direct ways. One of the roles which government plays is as a rule maker and in health care government lays down the rules under which the health market will operate. There is debate as to whether the rules inhibit innovations which might benefit patients, especially in relation to the pharmaceutical industry and presently in terms of technologies derived from advances in genetic science. It is not just the existence of rules which may be important but also how they are applied, ranging from universal prosecution for rule breaking, and infrequent prosecution, through to emphasis on voluntary compliance.

Government may require others to act in ways which they regard as meeting social objectives, including health care objectives. The identification of safety standards in employment may include employer provision of health care workers in the workplace in some industries. Government may require employers to pay sick leave and parental leave when children are ill. These are examples of government action which requires others to meet health objectives and for which government may or may not provide reimbursement. Government may also seek to encourage and stimulate others to act. This encouragement may take the form of information, education and exhortation or more direct action in which financial inducements or threats are used.

Another form of government action which has appeared in general social service provision in recent years is the contracting by government to other providers of services for which it has previously been responsible. In Britain, support services such as cleaning and laundering have been subject to contract or tender and the scope exists for more extensive contracting where government is a direct service provider, and these actions may have an impact on innovation.

The discussion of government action in relation to innovation in health care concluded with the observation that despite the very different histories of the health care systems in America and Britain the systems have become more alike over time rather than less alike. In Britain the establishment of a free universal health system has been modified by the growth of private health care insurance, private health care services and government taxation incentives to private health care producers and consumers. In America the federal government remains largely outside the realm of direct health care provision but has dramatically increased its financial contribution to funding health care. Alongside this growth of funding has come increasing government action to exert control and influence over the form and organization of health care provision. The organizational technologies in the two countries are still quite different but government actions have been more convergent than they have been divergent over the last fifty years.

Health care innovation and the long wave in economic activity

The literature concerning claimed links between the rate of technological innovation and long-wave cycles in economic activity which last about fifty to sixty years was briefly reviewed. The pattern of health care innovations across the four types of health care technology were identified and their timing examined from the beginning of the second long wave in 1843 to the middle of the fourth long wave in the 1970s.

The rate of innovation certainly seems to be lower during the recession phase of the long wave. Innovations are high in the depression phase, lending support to the argument that the depression may be a trigger for a wave of innovations which move economies out of the depression. However, the rate of innovation is also high through the recovery period and into the prosperity phases and this would support the view that innovations are pulled along by the increasing resources available as economic activity increases. This pattern of innovation would also suggest that capital spending in the health industry would be greatest from the initial upturn out of the depression through to the peak of the prosperity phase.

A number of tentative propositions were advanced concerning government action during the long wave and innovation. Government is a major provider of funding for health care whether it is a direct provider or not. Government income is likely to grow more rapidly during the prosperity and recession phases of the long wave than the depression and recovery phases. This proposition is based on various assumptions including that there exist time lags between investment in production technology and increases in company and personal incomes, that a progressive taxation structure is in place, and that inflation is part of the stagnation which occurs in the downswing of the long wave.

Government innovations in a service such as health care seem most likely to occur from the peak of the prosperity phase through to the initial part of the depression. The reasons for this are the availability of money for social expenditure stemming from the likely growth of government income at this time. The innovations that have occurred during the depression and recovery phases are more likely to have taken place outside the government sector, and the build up of these innovations may create opportunities for organizational innovations which maximize the potential benefits of innovations which have already been adopted. The pressure for political innovations may also take time to build as producer and consumer interests seek common ground in establishing issues in the political arena and identifying potential innovations in government policy. As the recession proceeds current government spending on health care may increase but that spending will be on minor organizational improvements which seek to extract the remaining benefits from existing technologies. Spending will also be oriented towards labour rather than capital because innovations which may require capital commitment are not available.

There is no suggestion that changes in health care technology are caused solely by long-term changes in the economy. Long waves in the economy are only one of many variables that must be included in any all-embracing theory. Links between variables are important to explore. Accounts of the welfare state have considered the impact of warfare, and wars do appear to have been a catalyst for action in relation to health care. Claimed links between the timing of wars and economic crises in the long wave provide one channel for drawing together these ideas with those concerning technological change.

ADDING TECHNOLOGY: AN INGREDIENT IN THE 'CUMU-LATIVE SYNTHESIS' OF KNOWLEDGE BUILDING ABOUT THE WELFARE STATE

This analysis of health care in Britain and America has sought to establish the proposition that an understanding of technology and how technology changes over time can contribute to our knowledge about the development of modern health care systems. The analysis has involved applying ideas and knowledge acquired from the examination of scientific knowledge, technology, and production and process innovations in industry, to the production of health care products and services. These 'imported' ideas have been used to reorder and re-evaluate the knowledge that we already have about the historical development of health care. In a sense new pieces have been added to the jigsaw and a contribution to the 'cumulative synthesis' of knowledge building about health care has been formulated. Whilst the analysis in Part I of this book can by no means be taken to document fully the role of technological change in the development of health care services the analysis is sufficiently well established to support the initial proposition that an understanding of technology and technological change has a valuable contribution to make in the process of knowledge building.

It could be argued that health care is peculiar amongst social services because of the relatively heavy usage of machine technologies and the emphasis on product innovations, especially in the pharmaceutical industry. Although other social services have not been examined in this book the general proposition that studies of technology and its development would assist in understanding these services is established in principle by the health care case study. It is not difficult to find evidence to support the relevance of this approach to other services. Education has used major elements of the factory system of organization in the classroom since the late nineteenth century. Bowles and Gintis

(1976, p. 224) have maintained that changes in the way education is structured have historically reflected changes in the manner in which production is structured in the economy in general. Broad innovations in publishing and printing have affected the ease of access and cost of learning materials. Advances in our knowledge about how people learn have been incorporated into the development of curricula and into teaching methods in the classroom. The advent of television and video communications have opened up new options for classroom learning and beyond the classroom in opening access to students far away from the physical educational institution. Computers are also transforming the amount of knowledge we can access as well as our systems of teaching. Even social security services have demonstrated that a changing technological base is of importance when seeking an appreciation of their development. Social insurance should be seen as part of the overall development of insurance-based services throughout national economies, in which new products and delivery technologies have been introduced. Hannah (1986, pp. 92–3) has described how employer and government pension schemes were modified in France, Britain and America in response to changing economic and social conditions. In effect new products were created as circumstances changed and this process can be seen in a similar light to the innovations of say Blue Shield and Blue Cross in health care in America. Social security has also been affected by innovations in general financial services, for instance, the methods of paying beneficiaries have been transformed many times by changes in the services and delivery mechanisms utilized by banks and other financial institutions. Systems of collecting, storing and updating information are critical to the effective operation of a social security system and advances in these technologies throughout the service and administrative sectors of an economy have had an impact on the technological base of social security. The case for adding the dimension of technological change to our analysis of all social service operations is clear. Some of the information necessary to generate a detailed account for the role of technology for social services other than health is available and could be pursued by interested researchers.

It has been implied in the discussion that historical changes in health care services may have had parallels in the development of other social services activities within the overall institutional framework of the welfare state. It might be argued that the value of a study of technology and technological change must be established for each social service before considering the contribution of technological change to an understanding of the welfare state as a whole. There are various reasons why this position is too restrictive and would ignore the opportunity at least to sketch out the questions that might be usefully pursued in future research. First the importance of health care production within both the total economy and as a major component of the welfare state has been clearly established. It is also worth noting that, in Britain at least, health care, along with education, are the two most widely supported and publicly recognized pillars of the welfare state. Second, whilst detailed studies of the impact of technological change on other social services are desirable, sufficient is already known to establish that technological change is an important factor even though it has not received systematic attention. Existing studies do indicate that similar factors to those in health will affect innovation and diffusion of innovations in these services too. Third, there are theoretical grounds for supporting the contribution which case studies can play in casting light on a wider picture. Raymond Boudon (1981, p. 92; 1986, p. 173) has emphasized that case studies and an analysis of different levels of activity are necessary to complement aggregate data. The study of health care in Part I provided a variety of levels of analysis of health care and conformed with Boudon's view that a substantial time scale is necessary to cast light on change processes. These pictures of health care also have value within Boudon's framework by illuminating changes in the wider structure of the welfare state.

INNOVATION AS A RESPONSE TO CRISIS IN THE WELFARE STATE

Uncertainty as the catalyst for innovation

The study of the effect of technological change on the development of health care appears to provide support for those who argue that uncertainty or perceived threat has been an important element in generating individual and community support for welfare state development. Goodin and Dryzak (1987) have used the notion of 'uncertainty' to address the question as to why people may support policies which aim to help the poor when they themselves are not poor. They examine this question with particular regard to the impact of war and conclude that uncertainties force people to consider the position of others and the possibility that they might find themselves in a similar position. Robert Morris (1986, p. 41) has followed a similar line of thought by linking changes in political structures, social organization and public policies to periods in which individuals, groups and national identity and tradition appear to be threatened. Threats may obviously stem from internal or external sources. Policies which acknowledge risk-sharing in the face of uncertainty or threat are thought likely to be more acceptable when the level of risk is high.

Looking at these questions in relation to health care the level of threat posed to an individual through illness may be perceived as a serious one, entailing the possibility of loss of functional capacity or even death. Given this level of perceived uncertainty for the individual it is not surprising that there is immense individual and public pressure on both health care producers and individual health care workers to provide all the care that is technologically feasible. The pressure to pursue every treatment is particularly intense in the face of health-threatening conditions which can affect large numbers of people, and whose incidence cannot be easily predicted. This response is also apparent in the financing of health care where in the American insurance-based system most people seek to cover all costs from the very first dollar rather than just large medical expenses. Fuchs (1986, pp. 298–9) explains this behaviour in terms of consumers wishing to remove the question of cost from decisions as to what health care they will utilize. They are removing money from the uncertainty equation even though from the viewpoint of economic rationality such behaviour appears to be ill-founded.

Uncertainty may be a catalyst for innovative activity in which the welfare state represents the expression of individual moral behaviour based upon risk-sharing as Goodin and Dryzek suggest. There are other interests which may motivate innovative action. Uncertainty may engender actions based upon appeals to national unity or preservation, or to collective solidarity amongst smaller groupings of people within society. Goodin and Dryzek do not refute this proposition but they do cast doubt upon it based upon an analysis of rationing behaviour in Britain during wartime. As they observe, however, Beveridge espoused ideas of national unity and sacrifice for the common good in the report which was to form the basis of the institutional reforms which laid the foundations of the contemporary welfare state in Britain. The mobilizing influence of an appeal to national pride and collective purpose within the community as a basis for postwar social reforms in Britain has received strong support from Barbara Wootton (1983). The discussion of technological change in health care has also indicated the importance of stimulating collective interest. Local community pride was mobilized effectively in the second half of the nineteenth century to fund local hospital provision. In general local and regional interests have had a role in achieving change in hospital care. Another example of collective action would be the operation of friendly societies which offered shared risk-taking based upon collective goals rather than just sharing of individual risks.

The discussion of the history of technological innovation in health care in this book has paid special attention to a particular source of uncertainty, namely the role which cyclical economic activity might have played in influencing the rate of technological innovation. Economic depressions have led to the questioning of the adequacy of existing social services and encouraged new ideas in health care and other services and the exploration of possible options for change. Berkowitz and McQuaid (1988), for example, argue that the 1920s depression led to a widespread questioning of the viability of the corporate-federal system of welfare that had emerged during the progressive era in America from around 1880 to 1920. Many corporate and community welfare schemes which were based on accumulating funds for use in an emergency were unable to cope with the demand for increased payments which took place in the 1930s. Quite simply the existing technology was seen to be inadequate (Berkowitz and McQuaid, 1988, p. 222).

The relationship between health care innovations and long-wave economic cycles was described in Chapter 5, and whilst the evidence neither clearly confirmed nor refuted the depression-trigger hypothesis the rate of innovation is at its greatest in the depression phase of the long wave. Health care historians have drawn many links between changes in health care and the influence of economic depression. Rosner (1979, p. 118) has described how philanthropic institutions declined in the wake of economic depression in the latter part of the nineteenth century. Markowitz and Rosner (1979, p. 186) claim that doctors acted to protect their jobs and incomes in the light of this depression, and again in the 1930s, by restricting entry to the profession through changing the requirements of training programmes. The introduction of Blue Cross and Blue Shield have been linked to the effect of the depression and entailed a substantial shift in public attitudes away from the previously established emphasis on the value of self-help and precautionary saving (Law, 1974, p. 6; Richardson, 1945).

Mensch's depression-trigger thesis for explaining technological innovation may not have received specific attention in the welfare state literature, but the onset of economic depressions has been frequently used to explain both the growth of government in industrial countries and seen as a contributing factor in the development of the modern welfare complex. Rothwell and Zegveld (1981) explain that 'periods of structural crisis in the economies of the industrial countries have been associated with the transformation of the role of the state' (p. 18). Economic depression during the late nineteenth century was followed by increasing government policy intervention in industrial economies. These actions included measures to regulate employer–labour relations, like defining who could work, the hours of work and physical conditions and safety requirements in the factory. After the depression of the 1920s and 1930s, acceptance of theories of central management of demand saw government in most industrial countries seek to regulate and plan their economies (Rimlinger, 1971). This growth in government bureaucracy has been linked to both economic depression and innovations in technology including specific management techniques (Erasaari, 1986).

The welfare state has been described as an institutional response to an economy based upon capitalism as the dominant mode of production. Welfare provisions can be seen as modifying class conflict which is implicit in a capitalist society and also responding to the effects of cyclical changes such as long waves which are inherent within a capitalist economy (Flora and Heidenheimer, 1981, pp. 22–3). The idea that economic depressions have stimulated discussion and subsequent development of individual social services and the welfare state as a whole has been frequently expressed. Bowles and Gintis (1976, pp. 224–34) relate changes in the structure of education in America to changes in economic structure which are presaged by depressions. Heclo (1981, pp. 384–5) has described the period after the depression of the 1870s and 1880s as one of great debate concerning policy issues and rapid legislative action covering many facets of social well-being, including social insurance programmes, changes in public education systems and developments in hospital organization. Similarly the depression of the 1930s and 1940s contributed to the surge of social legislation after the Second World War which put in place organizational innovations which laid down the structural features of contemporary welfare states. In general depressions have focused public attention on social policy questions and stimulated a level of public debate which does not occur at other times (Heclo, 1974, p. 286).

In Chapter 5 the links between economic depression and wars which may signal a future depression was noted. Warfare has been used to account for welfare state developments and the more general growth of government activity. Berkowitz and McQuaid (1988) have observed the rapid increase in government spending during wartime and the fact that spending does not return to prewar levels once hostilities cease. Wars are said to reveal past deficiencies in human services as reflected in the health and education status of both military and civilian populations. Educational standards, work skills and the health status of citizens are often scrutinized in wartime and found wanting. In relation to health care it was noted that the Boer War and the First World War both highlighted poor standards of health in Britain amongst recruits to the services. These concerns reflected back upon the adequacy of existing services including preventive health care provisions (Abbel-Smith, 1964, p. 284; Woodward, 1984, p. 75).

Wartime has also been characterized as a period when experimental techniques in services like health care can be tried given the severity of injuries and the reduction in effective regulatory oversight of health care practitioners. The Crimean War and American Civil War saw advances in both nursing and hospital care. America began industrial production of penicillin during the Second World War and the use of the drug to treat soldiers. In Britain the mental health service which emerged after the Second World War was influenced by an understanding of mental illnesses caused by stress. This understanding came about through attempts to treat soldiers who had experienced a variety of stress conditions during action (Jones, 1972, p. 270).

Economic depression and wartime represent threats to both national and individual security, but these are not the only sources of uncertainty. The history of health care is closely intertwined with the incidence of diseases which have threatened large numbers of people within a given country or amongst several countries. Typhoid, smallpox, tuberculosis, poliomyelitis, cancer, AIDS are just some of the more prominent examples of conditions which have caused fear throughout populations and have impacted upon health care research and services.

Threat to existing institutions can also come from the pursuit of group interests which it is feared might be pursued through physical violence. Marxist accounts of the welfare state in capitalist countries portray the welfare state as a means by which class conflict is mediated and the working class is 'bought off' by material provisions in social services (Miliband, 1969). Whilst the more overt discrimination of the Poor Law divisions between the deserving and undeserving has been abolished by the modern welfare state, the tools of 'means-testing' or 'targeting' can fulfil a similar purpose in identifying an underclass and creating internal distinctions in the response in welfare systems to the working class. A threat to existing institutions is also present in most industrial countries because of ethnic divisions within the population. Racial violence has been used to explain the introduction of welfare state policies which benefit specific ethnic groups (Isaac and Kelly, 1981). Another source of uncertainty is the interaction between population changes and social policy provisions. The history of the modern welfare state is of an expansion by social service programmes to cover an increasing proportion of national populations. Educational provisions have been expanded to include children at a younger age and extended to increase the age of compulsory school attendance and encourage higher retention into tertiary education programmes. The history of health care in both Britain and America is also one of opening access to health care to increasingly larger sections of the population. The impact of demographic changes such as increased longevity on the availability and funding of a wide variety of social services is a major source of uncertainty in contemporary policy debate on the future of the welfare state.

Events which generate uncertainty within social institutions as perceived by significant numbers of the population and which are also seen as a threat to the security of individuals are likely to stimulate debate about social policy. The source of uncertainty may be externally or internally generated. The history of the welfare state and of an individual service such as health care is at least partially a description of responses evoked by such debates. This is not to argue that innovations in health care, or the welfare state as a whole, are determined by the demand to defuse uncertainty. Uncertainty is a catalyst for debate about the efficacy of present actions because what is actually happening, as opposed to what was thought to be happening, frequently becomes apparent and discussed. A climate is created in which change, including innovation in the technological base of the welfare state, is debated and new options identified. As was explained in Chapter 1 some innovations may be grounded in existing structures and constructions of the problem but others will represent a break or 'mutation' from existing perceptions (Boudon, 1986, pp. 167–8).

The motivation for change in the welfare state has roots other than individual and collective moral behaviour generated by uncertainty and these were also considered in the discussion of technological innovation and production of health care in Part I of this book. The welfare state consists of technologies which are utilized to produce goods and services. The market for those goods and services may be different because of government involvement as a producer, as a funder of provision and consumption, and as an extensive regulator of the market. Welfare state activities are not entirely unique in these respects, however. Social service production is an economic process and the reasons for innovation will have some communality with those for the production of other goods and services. The adoption and diffusion of innovation will be influenced by an assessment of the rate of return on investment and the degree of risk involved. Assessment of innovations in social services will be modified by the particular characteristics of the social service production, but as in other areas of activity risk and rate of return will be important influences on producer behaviour. The influence of uncertainty in all its facets will be incorporated into the assessments which producers make.

The attitudes of workers towards innovation are influential in a service such as health care where professional socialization prizes highly scientific advances in knowledge and technology. The ascribing of status between and within health care occupational groups is partially a reflection of the acquisition and utilization of new technologies. Individually and collectively, workers in health care have a strong self-interest in promoting innovations which are valued within their occupations. The power of labour within health care and in other areas of the welfare state, which is often strongly professionalized, presents a barrier to innovations which substitute for labour or challenge worker control in other ways. Indeed the position of labour in health and social service production in general could be seen as evidence of the gradual establishment of economic dualism in industrial economies. Economic dualism occurs when segments of the labour force become insulated from uncertainty and variable demand for their services (Berger and Piore, 1980). Workers' needs in this situation in effect become incorporated into the planning and decision-making process such as innovation in much the same manner as capital requirements. Threats to the position of labour, such as economic depression, could affect the level of return to labour in the form of wages and salaries. Various illustrations have been described of the ways in which workers in health care have sought to counteract this kind of threat to their position.

Crisis and the welfare state

The 1970s and 1980s have seen widespread criticism of the operation and future viability of the welfare state. Criticisms have come from many diverse perspectives, including the political right and left. Criticisms have been increasingly strongly expressed since the early 1960s. During the last twenty years these criticisms, combined with concerns about the level of economic performance in industrial countries, have placed debate about the welfare state in a central position for discussion amongst policy makers. The widespread concern amongst industrial countries has been evident in international conferences such as the conference organized by the Organization for Economic Development and Cooperation in Paris in 1981 (OECD, 1981). Just as policy makers have focused on the operation of the welfare state, so the general population with direction from the mass media has also been encouraged to ask similar questions.

The reasons for concern about the future of the welfare state have been well documented elsewhere (in Friedman and Friedman, 1980; Gough, 1979; Mishra, 1984; Offe, 1984, for example) and will only be summarized briefly here. Debate is essentially focused around three central issues: first the effectiveness of the welfare state and individual social services in achieving their objectives, second the resource cost of the operation of the welfare state, and finally the validity and desirability of the values and objectives being pursued.

Effectiveness

Similar questions are raised about the welfare state as a whole as about individual social services. These questions include:

- Does the service work in the sense of achieving the objectives which have been identified?
- Do those in most need receive the service or do other consumers and vested interests amongst providers of services gain effective control over resources?
- Do service workers including professional and bureaucratic elites have too much power in both policy formulation and implementation?
- Does government intervention and regulation in reality improve the welfare of the population as a whole?

These kinds of concerns have been apparent in the debate about the effectiveness of modern health care systems. Attention has been paid to the impact of health care services on the level of illness within the community. The focus has, however, increasingly been changed to question the impact of health care on the quality of health and whether health status has been significantly improved within the total population and within those sections of the population whose health status is most at risk. These questions about the effectiveness of health care services also raise doubts about the value of many technologies used in the production of services. The power which health care producers and health care workers exert relative to consumers has been strongly criticized. This power is viewed as being reinforced and sanctioned by government through its role in regulating the labour market in health care and thereby legitimating professional power. The ability of government to act as an efficient provider or funder of health care has also been widely questioned and alternatives advocated.

Cost

In the late 1960s and 1970s many countries in the OECD experienced the combination of rapid growth in public expenditure combined with sharply reduced or even negative rates of economic growth. Associated with these changes has been the generation of substantial imbalances in national budgets. Welfare state expenditures during this period have tended to grow more rapidly than all other forms of public spending. This has helped focus public attention and debate on the way in which resources are used through government social expenditures. Increases in social expenditure have been partly generated by government policies which have extended the coverage for particular social services within the population and by demographic changes which have increased the usage of particular service programmes. An example of these kinds of effects would be the impact which ageing within the populations of many industrialized countries has had upon the costs of income support and health care programme costs.

The future economic viability of specific programmes and services and the whole welfare state appears open to question within the much wider context of how to manage government budgets and national debt. The tendency for the burden of taxation upon individuals and companies to increase is claimed seriously to impair the incentives to generate individual and corporate income. Low rates of economic growth are said to reflect a growing imbalance between public and private sector resource use. Resources used in private sector production of goods and services are portrayed as growth generating whilst public spending in general and social spending in particular are not.

Values and objectives

The extension of the institutions of the welfare state to provide broadly based services available throughout the population has been criticized as an abandonment of the original goals of the welfare state. These goals are said to have emphasized the aim to assist those in greatest need and ensure that poverty and disease are effectively combated in relatively affluent societies. Welfare systems are criticized for apparently abandoning these goals and using resources on those who do not really need help. Detailed analyses of specific services and programmes are used to demonstrate that middle-class and sometimes wealthy people capture the benefits of social service programmes and that those in most need may still remain in relative poverty. The growth of the welfare state was part of the wider growth of government in industrialized societies. The centralization of power within government political and bureaucratic institutions has been seen as restricting economic and individual freedoms. Whilst arguing from very different perspectives, critics from the 'new right' and the political left have both advocated reduction in the power exercised by the centralized institutions of the state. In relation to the welfare state these pressures have been manifest in demands for privatization and contracting of services on the one hand and devolution and decentralization in the organizational structures of services on the other.

Progress

It could be argued that the problems which seem present in the contemporary welfare state are merely a reflection of a much broader questioning of the relationship between science, technology and progress. Our perception of technology and technological change has been closely related to the much wider concept of 'progress' or 'enlightenment'. Robert Nisbet (1980) says that our idea of progress 'holds that mankind has advanced in the past ... is now advancing and will continue to advance through the foreseeable future' (pp. 5–6). This view of progress rests on two main propositions. The first proposition is that the accretion of knowledge over time, especially scientific knowledge and its application to technology, allows increasing control over the natural and mechanical world. The second proposition is that this control generates increasing material welfare and an improvement in man's moral and spiritual condition which is then translated into higher moral standards and aesthetic tastes (Almond *et al.*, 1982, pp. 1–15; Nisbet, 1980, p. 6). The idea of progress has been taken to imply a continual improvement in the human condition over time and a clear belief that the world of 'tomorrow' will be better than the world of 'today'. It is true that there may be periods in which stagnation or even regression may occur, but these are seen as essentially minor fluctuations in the movement towards a more perfect end state which will eventually embrace all humanity. It is the generation of knowledge, and especially scientific knowledge, which is the catalyst of progress and this knowledge is derived from human reason rather than divine revelation. Technological development and the economic growth which it generates are the means by which material and moral well-being will be enhanced.

An acceptance of the idea of progress has been embedded into the evolution of the welfare state and alongside it certain assumptions about the potential capacity of technology in the social and political world. These assumptions have been of particular importance in the following areas.

Social science

The dominant concept of progress implies that the natural, physical and mechanical worlds can be understood and harnessed through the pursuit of scientific inquiry. The development of the social sciences, especially since the nineteenth century, has been seen as offering the similar potential capacity to chart our social environment. This understanding of the social world would enable social problems to be understood and techniques to be developed in such a manner as to allow social processes to be controlled and social problems to be resolved. This belief is well illustrated by the responses to the influential social surveys of poverty in late Victorian England by Booth and Rowntree. These surveys were seen by many as holding out the promise that poverty could be 'isolated' and 'cured' in a similar manner to the way in which medical science had cured cholera or typhoid (Rose, 1972, pp. 33–4). Similar ideas about the susceptibility of a wide range of social problems to social science was apparent in America during the same period and Leiby refers to these developments as 'scientific philanthropy' (1978, pp. 90–110).

Just as the natural sciences have been viewed as not just important in themselves but also in generating practical benefits to society, so the social sciences have been perceived as a powerful potential force for social betterment. This force for betterment has found partial expression in the policies and institutional arrangements of the welfare state. Rule (1978, p. 3) has described how this faith in the potential of social science has been assimilated into public expectations about the possible effectiveness of social policy interventions. This belief in the potential of social science and its application by professional technicians in the services of health, education, social security and community social services has been closely linked with the historical development of the welfare state and especially with the rapid expansion in institutions and programmes from the late 1930s onwards.

The growth of government

The development of welfare states has been associated with changing views about the general role which government should play in society. Wildavsky (1982) has identified five distinguishing features of the growth in the size and scope of government from the nineteenth century to the present day: first its size, historically, in comparison to the private sector, second its size in absolute terms in comparison to the past, third the growth in the number of government programmes, fourth the increasing diversity in government activity, and finally the effect of government on people's lives.

Alongside the growth of government has been the development of a 'policy science' which seeks to identify the critical elements in public policy decisions and to provide rational techniques which can be applied to the decision-making process. Bell (1976) has described the emergence of policy science as part of a wider process of social control: 'every modern society now lives by innovation and social control of change and tries to anticipate the future in order to plan ahead. This commitment to social control introduces the need for planning and forecasting into society' (p. 20). Social policy making in the public arena is accordingly the subject of attempts to forecast future changes and, through increasingly complex decision-making techniques, produce planned responses to those changes. Contemporary questioning of the composition and future of the welfare state seldom appears to depart from the belief that the issues being confronted are potentially capable of solution by the technologies of policy analysis and implementation.

Social values

The claimed links between economic growth, knowledge and the improvement of the human condition have been stated clearly in Kumar's description of the post-industrial ideal:

> It sees in the extension of science, the application of ever more sophisticated and complex technology, and the growth of services, the indications of an increasingly prosperous, civilized and knowledgeable society. It is a society capable – thanks to scientific knowledge and scientific management – of more or less continuous material growth, which in turn makes possible the realization of a service society, suffused with an ethos of social responsibility, social welfare and the service ideal. (Kumar, 1978, pp. 242–43).

It is the problem of scarcity, and poverty associated with scarcity, which has been described as the central threat to human well-being in developing countries since the Middle Ages (Rimlinger, 1971). The social policy response to poverty prior to the late nineteenth century was based on the relief, and

not removal, of poverty and instituting social control mechanisms to prevent any threat of rebellion. The twin uncertainties
of cyclical activity in an emerging capitalist economy and the
potential threat of an urbanized and impoverished group of
workers have been described as important factors in the development of welfare states. This was apparent, for example, in the
debate about the 'social question' in Germany which preceded
the introduction of social insurance in the late nineteenth century
(Ritter, 1986). The development of a welfare infrastructure in
industrial countries has become more extensive over time. The
welfare state offers what Gellner (1987, p. 100) has referred to
as 'protection against vulnerability'. It is a form of protection
which has been extended from a relatively small residual section
of the population in the nineteenth century to almost universal
coverage during the course of the twentieth century.

The pursuit of security, protection and social justice through
the welfare state rests on the assumption that it is reasonable
to expect continuing economic growth driven by technological innovation, and that: 'Affluence thus offers humanity the
very chance of humane behaviour that had been obviated too
often in the past by physical scarcity' (a position attributed
to Gellner in Hall, 1981, p. 198). Planning the distribution
of an expanding 'cake' allows painful choices between con-
flicting values and claims to be largely avoided. As Flora
(1985, p. 13) suggests, the welfare state has become an increasingly visible channel for the distribution and stabilization of
the life chances of the whole of the population. Alongside
the pervasiveness of the welfare state is the belief held by
many that the constituent policies and institutions of welfare are based upon either a broad social consensus, or at
least tacit assent, around the values which should be pursued.

Not all commentators, however, share this view of the welfare
state as an expression of social cohesion. Gellner (1987) refers
to economic growth as creating what he terms the 'Danegeld
Fund' and the welfare state as one of the major drawers on this
fund whereby '[if] you can bribe most of the people most of
the time, it may be possible to relax the more brutal traditional
methods of ensuring social conformity' (p. 15). Welfare states
can thus be seen as promising material gain to large sections
of the population through social policies and programmes.

The second part of Gellner's statement about social control is also important. The scope of government monitoring and regular interventions in the lives of individuals and groups is substantially expanded through the welfare state. Social service programmes operate within what Kumar refers to as 'the therapeutic mode' (1978, p. 196) in which the assessment and treatment of individuals, in the context of their living group, is a central feature of the service process. Donzelot (1980) has described the emergence of the 'psy' occupations, which control the therapeutic mode, during the latter part of the last century. These professional groups lay claim to knowledge derived from both medical and social sciences and Donzelot describes the complex web of mechanisms which is wound around individuals and families in the name of publicly sanctioned 'caring' services. The question as to whether Kumar's 'ethos of social responsibility' stems from convergence over the values which should underpin social services or the employment of subtle, and not so subtle, mechanisms of social control is very much open to debate.

Religion and secularization

An important factor in any discussion of progress is the proposition that the position of a divine agency as the source of knowledge and authority has been replaced by a belief that knowledge is created and marshalled through human reason. Gellner (1987, p. 16) says that a belief in the continual critical evaluation of our knowledge of the world around us contrasts with an approach to knowledge based on religious doctrine in which status, ritual and moral values underpin a firm world vision.

Historically, religious organizations have played an important role in influencing social policy and the provision of social services. It appears that over a long period of time, and especially since the nineteenth century, churches have been displaced as the major providers of welfare. They have become providers of specialist services which complement the main forms of service provision which come directly or indirectly through government. Although we may not have a detailed analysis of the secularization of social policy (Higgins, 1981, p.

96), there are many accounts of welfare in different countries which cast light on the process (see Donzelot, 1980; Morris, 1986; Roberts, 1979, for example). Higgins (1981, p. 92) says that there are two main explanations for the secularization of welfare in the literature. First, the effects of industrialization and urbanization mean that it is no longer viable to have a geographically localized welfare system. Coherence of the whole system and wider coverage become increasingly important to the growth of the welfare state. Second, religion no longer exerts the necessary level of control within society and the activities of organized religion such as alms giving endanger the success of government-provided or -controlled welfare services. Education policy has been one of the main battlegrounds between church and government in the move to secularization. That education should be the centre of debate is not unexpected given the dominant explanations of progress and social change. Industrialization involves an increasingly complex division of labour and requires a formally educated labour force (Kerr, 1983, p. 6). Progress dictates the acceptance of continual occupational mobility (Gellner, 1987, p. 15) and social mobility (a position attributed to Dahrendorf in Hall, 1981, p. 136) and education is the key to creating an environment in which these conditions are met. In most industrial countries church control over the institutions of education and the content of what is learnt has passed from the church to the state.

A much harder question to answer is what influence religious ideas and beliefs have upon social policy and welfare systems. The values which might guide human behaviour derived from the major world religions such as care, concern, mercy, benevolence and so on are to be found in the formal language of the secular welfare state. The rationale for subscribing to such values is however no longer based upon religious belief when translated into the written language of policy documents and government legislation.

Alongside the growth of the welfare state has been the emergence of professional and semi-professional occupational groups employed to provide social services. Some writers have explored the argument that such workers represent the modern secular equivalents of religious priests within churches in the way that they construct and sustain belief systems for themselves and those they serve (Halmos, 1965; North, 1972). What is less clear is to what extent religious belief represents a major motivating factor in occupational choice in these professions and how religious belief and knowledge derived from natural and social sciences are reconciled in the actions of these workers.

It could be argued that the questioning of the future viability of the welfare state mirrors much more fundamental concerns about the capacity of science and technology to contribute positively to human well-being. The links between the ideals of the welfare state and ideas of progress and enlightenment in modern societies have been briefly described above. Progress has been seen in the past as being firmly grounded in the knowledge derived from scientific endeavour. This knowledge can be harnessed through technology to gain increasing control over the physical and natural world and to generate material well-being. Material well-being enables humanity to pursue moral goals in which not only material well-being but also emotional and spiritual goals are achievable. Science, including the social sciences, can yield knowledge and techniques which allow for the management of relations between people within societies and between societies. The welfare state has been seen as an expression of this belief that individual and social well-being are susceptible to scientific endeavour. The human condition can be enhanced in relation to both material and moral goals.

The crisis in the welfare state could be seen as merely part of a wider questioning of this concept of progress and the central position of knowledge and scientific endeavour in the achievement of progress. There are obvious concerns about the impact which specific technologies have on humanity and our environment both now and in the future. The development of environmental politics during the last twenty years and the emergence of 'green' political parties in Europe and elsewhere is evidence of these concerns. Whilst there may be a growing acceptance of the need for controls and indeed the desirability of abolishing the use of specific technologies it seems unlikely that there will be any widespread abandonment of science and technology as the basis of knowledge generation and application. The adoption of more controls and greater caution about the possible impacts of technologies does not in itself seem to herald a major reformulation of our ideas of progress. The crisis in the welfare state is therefore not likely to indicate a widespread turning away from a belief in the potential which knowledge generation and technologies in both social and physical sciences have to enhance human welfare. It seems much more likely to be described as a period in which existing technologies, including organizational technologies, have been exhausted and the search is going on for new technologies which will open up fresh possibilities in the production and distribution of social services.

'Crisis' in the welfare state and cycles in economic activity

The exploration of technological innovation in health care and the relationship of innovation to cycles in economic activity can shed some light on the debate about a 'crisis' in the welfare state. In Chapter 5 a series of tentative propositions were advanced concerning the rate and form of technological innovations in the welfare state during different phases of the long wave. These propositions are based upon the analysis of innovation in health care technology since the mid-nineteenth century. What is being asserted is that certain events are more likely to occur at specified points in the long wave than at other points. It should be remembered, however, that there are many other factors involved which may modify the observed pattern of innovation.

Depression/recovery phases

Basic innovations Radical new technologies will be introduced during these phases. These technologies will include innovations specific to the particular social services within the welfare state and technologies drawn from other areas of production. Where innovations are drawn from outside the welfare state there may be a time lag in adoption before the potential of such innovations is recognized. Especially important will be those innovations which constitute the infrastructure generated by the cluster of technologies which underpin the long wave. The time lag involved may move the adoption of the innovation towards the recovery/prosperity phase of the long wave.

Labour   Measures will be introduced to meet the labour requirements of the new technologies and government will play a special role in the training of workers in the social services. Government has a longstanding position as a provider of professional training for social service workers and as the sanctioning body for recognition of both a profession and the individual worker.

Capital spending   Capital spending rather than current expenditure is likely to be higher during these phases of the long wave than at other points. Available theories of long-wave activity would all support this proposition. The depression-trigger and prosperity-pull theories would identify these phases as being characterized by high levels of innovation, and innovations commonly require capital spending on plant and equipment. Theories based upon capital availability and commitment, such as that put forward by Mandel (1983) which indicates that capital accumulates during the course of the long wave and cannot be invested for an acceptable rate of return during the downswing and Forrester's (1983) theory that capital commitment begins in the upswing and is transmitted throughout the economy by a multiplier effect, would both indicate accelerating capital spending during the upswing of the long wave. Capital spending in the welfare state may be concentrated in the initial upswing of the long wave from the base of the depression through to the early stages of recovery.

Recovery/prosperity phases

Basic and improvement innovations   The introduction of new technologies will continue through these phases with changes both to the content of social services and the processes through which they are made available to consumers. Basic innovations which have been introduced are modified by a flow of improvement innovations which seek to realize the potential benefits of those innovations.

Labour   The balance between capital and labour spending may change during this stage of the long wave. The welfare state is an important employer of professional, managerial and, in the case of health services, technical labour. The state has usually contributed to the initial training of this labour force and to continuing training which is seen as necessary for the maintenance of its effectiveness. Dual labour market proponents argue that labour in modern industrial economies becomes segmented into two groups, one group which is likely to have continuing employment security irrespective of economic conditions and the other group for whom employment is highly sensitive to overall economic activity. Labour in the welfare state is likely to form part of that section of the labour force which dual labour market theorists (Berger and Piore, 1980) claim has acquired the ability to insulate itself against uncertainty and variation in the level of demand. The strength of this section of the labour force is such that its requirements are increasingly incorporated into planning and decision-making systems. In return for lessened vulnerability to changes in demand this section of the labour force must accept that it will be expected to respond to continuing technological innovation (Gellner, 1987). The socialization of professional workers in health care enshrines these expectations in the value systems of those workers. Professional labour in general and as evidenced in the welfare state has acquired some of the characteristics of capital in that a large and continuing investment has been made in its preparation and maintenance. Innovation has become viewed as being dependent on the generation and application of knowledge which is at least partly controlled and fostered by professional labour. During these phases of the long wave the balance of spending in welfare state activities between capital and labour will tend to shift towards labour spending as labour is prepared and employed to realize the innovations becoming available. In social service production, such as health services, innovations have frequently been labour enhancing rather than providing an opportunity for labour substitution.

Prosperity/recession phases

Basic and improvement innovations The flow of basic innovations continues at least until the peak of the long wave and improvement innovations become more numerous.

Government innovation It is during the prosperity phase that major innovations in government policy towards service production within the welfare state are most likely to occur. The flow of innovations which have appeared during the upswing of the long wave are interacting with the technologies which are still being used and developed from previous long waves. Government has the opportunity to produce organizational innovations which will facilitate the potential gains from this innovation flow.

Labour Spending on labour relative to capital tends to increase and the rate of innovation diminishes after the peak of the long wave and as increases in government income feed through into social expenditure.

Recession/depression phases

Basic and improvement innovations The flow of innovations diminishes sharply and improvement innovations no longer offer significant gains. The effectiveness and cost of existing technologies tend to come under some scrutiny.

Government innovation Government is less likely to introduce major new innovations of its own during this period. Continued buoyancy in government income combined with the extensions in social service programme coverage that frequently accompany the innovations which government has made during the prosperity phase mean that social spending is likely to continue to grow for much of this period. It is only when the depression becomes established that the efficacy of current technologies and the public cost of sustaining social service programmes comes under careful scrutiny.

Labour In the absence of new sources of innovation and with government income and programme coverage having been extended spending on labour is likely to remain high. The questioning of the power and cost of labour will not tend to occur until the depression is firmly established.

Technological innovations and improvement innovations have a limited life span. They may diffuse at different rates within an industry or between countries but they all tend to follow an 'S' curve of some kind in which a point is reached where the potential benefits of the innovation have been largely realized. All long-wave theorists agree, albeit for different reasons, that there will be a considerable reduction in the rate of innovation during the downswing of the long wave and that this is part of the wider picture of economic stagnation in national and international economies. Important basic and improvement innovations have taken place earlier in the long wave, and organizational innovations, especially government innovations, have been introduced by the prosperity phase. The increased value which can be extracted from labour in the face of low levels of innovation has limits even in relatively labour-intensive service industries. Peitchin's (Rothwell and Zegveld, 1981, pp. 222–7) research confirms this view that the present potential of labour in service activities has been more or less fully realized through improvement in the quality of labour, and the scope for employment growth is restricted in the absence of innovation.

Flora and Heidenheimer (1981) have referred to the role of stagnation in the development of crisis in the welfare state: 'The modern welfare state was a product of capitalism. If the earning and learning capacities of capitalism are entering a phase of stagnation, then the limits of welfare state development may become apparent through a series of crises' (p. 31). The welfare state encompasses a multitude of technologies which are used to generate the goods and services which the welfare state provides. These technologies include organizational technology within which production is structured and in which government plays a critical role. Chandler (Hummon, 1984) argues that technological advances in production generate changes in the scale of production which make it necessary for innovations in organizational technologies to also be introduced. This view has been supported in the analysis of health care technology with organizational innovations by producers and government following rather than preceding other kinds of innovation. These organizational forms will remain subject to only minor modifications as long as the production technologies which stimulated them remain viable. Many technologies will be diffused between industrial countries. As the technological base in different countries tends to converge in the face of diffusion, and stagnation in the rate of innovation occurs, then organizational technologies in different countries will equally tend to converge over time, all other things being equal. The contrast between the organization of American and British health care systems provides some support for this view. It has been argued that the organizational environment in the two countries has tended to converge rather than diverge in the face of economic stagnation.

The notion of crisis in the welfare state can be seen as a reflection of the lifespan of the technological base of its service activities. Innovations flowed from the depression of the 1920s and 1930s and through to the prosperity phase from the late 1940s to the mid-1960s. Government innovations which have laid down the institutional framework of the modern welfare state have their roots in the prosperity phase. It appears that an important but neglected dimension of the contemporary crisis in the welfare state is the impact of stagnation on technological innovation during the downswing of the long wave. This stagnation is accomppanied by questioning of the adequacy and appropriateness of existing technologies including the welfare state as the expression of existing organizational technologies. Morris (1986, p. 41) describes this process as initially a 'conservative tide' looking to the past which will subsequently be followed by a search for new technologies and policy reforms for the future.

It is not possible to foresee what the radical innovations are which will underpin the fifth long-wave economic cycle. The work of 'future watchers' such as Toffler (1980) indicate that it is innovations in communications and information storage and analysis which will transform production, especially the production of services. Work may no longer be tied to a specific location in the office or the factory and may be partially home-based. If the infrastructure is created to realize some of those technologies which are already in existence then the work of Gershuny (1983a; 1983b) and Blackburn (1985) would indicate that major changes in health care and education could follow. Some types of health care could be transferred back into the home and software packages might allow distance monitoring of personal health and illness. The 'crisis' may lead to substitution of capital for labour in health care and other social services such as education in ways that have not been possible in the past. These types of innovation would also have an important impact on other social services such as income support programmes and throughout the personal and community services sectors.

The debate about the future of the welfare state allows us to re-evaluate the past emphasis on seeing social services and policies as a distributional mechanism alone. As Taylor–Gooby (1983) has pointed out, a myopic focus on distribution ignores the reality that for most people the only way in which their position can be improved is through advances in production. Gershuny (1983a; 1985) has demonstrated how new technologies in the form of consumer durables have effectively transformed the capacity of households to produce goods and services. In many areas of production innovations such as these have not only changed the mode of production for the household but also reordered access to goods and services. The effect of these kinds of innovations has been to equalize access to a wide range of goods and services between the rich and the poor although the form of the goods and services may be transformed in the process. Perhaps it is consumer durables which will change future social service production and open up new options for redistribution policies.

There is likely to be a time lag between innovations in service production technologies such as these and organizational changes which provide the institutional framework for social service provision. The major organizational innovations which will transform the institutional framework of the welfare state may not be introduced until well into the next century. Only then will the possibilities for new technologies in social services be more clearly established and debates about the technical, commercial and political feasibility of such changes be resolved. The period of 'crisis', uncertainty and debate about future options is likely to be with us for some considerable time yet.

References

Abbott, L. F. (1976), *Social Aspects of Innovation and Industrial Technology*, Department of Industry CFIT Paper No. 1 (London: HMSO).

Abel-Smith, B. (1964), *The Hospitals 1800–1948* (London: Heinemann).

Abel-Smith, B. (1976), *Value for Money in Health Services. A Comparative Study* (London: Heinemann).

Aldcroft, D. H. (1983), *The British Economy Between the Wars* (London: Philip Allen).

Almond, G. A., Chodorow, M. and Pearce, R. H. (eds.) (1982), *Progress and its Discontents*, (Berkeley, Calif.: University of California Press).

Altenstetter, C. (ed.) (1981), *Innovation in Health Policy and Service Delivery. A Cross National Perspective* (Konigstein: Oelgeshlager, Gunn & Hain).

Altman, S. H. and Wallack, S. S. (1979), 'Is medical technology the culprit behind rising health costs? The case for and against', in Proceedings of the 1977 Sun Valley Forum on National Health Care, op. cit., pp. 24–38.

Armour, P. K. (1981), *The Cycles of Social Reform. Mental Health Policy Making in the United States, England and Sweden* (Washington, DC.: University Press of America).

Armstrong, D. (1983), *Political Anatomy of the Body. Medical Knowledge in the Twentieth Century* (Cambridge: Cambridge University Press).

Ascher, K. (1987), *The Politics of Privatization. Contracting Out Public Services* (London: Macmillan).

Ashford, D. (1986), *The Emergence of the Welfare States* (Oxford: Blackwell).

Baker, J. (1979), 'Social conscience and social policy', *Journal of Social Policy*, vol. 8, no. 2, pp. 177–206.

Banta, D. (1981), 'Public policy and medical technology: critical issues reconsidered', in Altenstetter, op. cit., pp. 57–85.

Bean, P. and MacPherson, S. (eds.) (1983), *Approaches to Welfare* (London: Routledge & Kegan Paul).

Bell, D. (1976), *The Coming of Post-Industrial Society* (Harmondsworth: Penguin).

Benson, I. and Lloyd, J. (1983), *New Technology and Industrial Change* (London/New York: Kogan Page/Nicholls).

Berger, S. and Piore, M. J. (1980), *Dualism and Discontinuity in Industrial Societies* (Cambridge: Cambridge University Press).

Berkowitz, E. D. and McQuaid, K. (1988), *Creating the Welfare State: The Political Economy of Twentieth Century Reform*, 2nd edn (New York: Praeger).

Bice, T. W. (1981), 'Regulation of capital investments of hospitals in the United States: certificate of need controls', in Altenstetter, op. cit., pp. 43–54.

Birenbaum, A. (1981), *Health Care and Society* (Montclair, NJ.: Allenhead/Osmun).

Blackburn, P., Coombs, R. and Green, K. (1985), *Technology, Economic Growth and the Labour Process* (London: Macmillan).

Blume, S. (1981), 'Technology in medical diagnosis: aspects of its dynamic and impact', in Altenstetter, op. cit., pp. 107–24.

Boserup, E. (1981), *Population and Technological Change* (Chicago: University of Chicago Press).

Boudon, R. (1981), *The Logic of Social Action* (London: Routledge & Kegan Paul).

Boudon, R. (1986), *Theories of Social Change* (Cambridge: Polity).

Boulding, K. (1981), *Evolutionary Economics* (Beverly Hills, Calif.: Sage).

Boulding, K. (ed.) (1984), *The Economics of Social Betterment* (London: Macmillan).

Bowles, S. and Gintis, H. (1976), *Schooling in Capitalist America* (London: Routledge & Kegan Paul).

Boyle, C., Wheale, P. and Surgess, B. (1985), *People, Science and Technology. A Guide to Advanced Industrial Society* (Brighton: Wheatsheaf).

Brada, J. C. (1980), 'Government policy and the transfer of pharmaceutical technology among developed countries', in Helms, op. cit., pp. 37–53.

Braun, H. G., Laumer, H., Leibfritz, W. and Sherman, H. C. (eds.) (1983), *The European Community in the 1980s* (Munich/Aldershot: Institute for Economic Research/Gower).

Brooks, H. (1982), 'Social and technological innovation', in Lundstedt and Colglazier, op. cit., pp. 2–35.

Browning, R. (1986), *Politics and Social Welfare Policy in the United States* (Knoxville, Tenn.: University of Tennessee Press).

Carrier, J. and Kendall, I. (1973), 'Social policy and social change', Journal of Social Policy, vol. 2, no. 2, pp. 209–34.

Cartwright, F. F. (1977), *A Social History of Medicine* (New York: Longman).

Central Health Services Council, Ministry of Health (1963), *The Field Work of the Family Doctor* Gillie, Report (London: HMSO).

Chapman, S. (1974), *Jessie Boot of Boots the Chemists* (London: Hodder & Stoughton).

Clark, J., Freeman, C. and Soete, L. (1983), 'Long waves, inventions and innovations', in Freeman, op. cit., pp. 63–77.

Consultative Council on Medical and Allied Services of the Ministry of Health (1920), *The Report of the Consultative Council*, Dawson Report (London: HMSO).

Delbeke, J. (1983), 'Recent long-wave theories: a critical survey', in Freeman, op. cit., pp. 1–12.

Donzelot, J. (1980), *Policing of Families: Welfare Versus the State* (London: Hutchinson).

van Duijn, J. J. (1983), *The Long Wave in Economic Life* (London: Allen & Unwin).

Eisenstadt, S. N. and Ahimer, O. (eds.) (1985), *The Welfare State and Its Aftermath* (London: Croom Helm).

Ellis, A. and Kumar, K. (eds.) (1983), *Dilemmas of Liberal Democracies. Studies in Fred Hirsch's Social Limits of Growth* (London: Tavistock).

Erasaari, E. (1986), 'The new social state?', *Acta Sociologica*, vol. 29, no. 3, pp. 225–41.

Evans, E. J. (1983), *The Forging of the Modern State Early Industrial Britain 1783–1870* (London: Longman).

Feldstein, P. J. (1979), *Health Care Economics* (New York: Wiley).

Flora, P. (1985), 'On the history and current problems of the welfare state', in Eisenstadt and Ahimer, op. cit., pp. 11–30.

Flora, P. and Heidenheimer, A. J. (eds.) (1981a), *The Development of the Welfare States in Europe and America* (London: Transaction Books).

Flora, P. and Heidenheimer, A. J. (1981b), 'The historical core and changing boundaries of the welfare state', in Flora and Heidenheimer, op. cit., pp. 17–34.

Forrester, J. W. (1977), 'Growth cycles', *De Economist*, vol. 125, pp. 525–43.

Forrester, J. W. (1983), 'Innovation and economic change', in Freeman, op. cit., pp. 126–34.

Freeman, C. (1982), *The Economics of Industrial Innovation* (London: Frances Pinter).

Freeman C. (ed.) (1983), *Long Waves in the World Economy* (London: Butterworths).

Freeman, C., Clark, J. A. and Soete, L. L. G. (1982), *Unemployment and Technical Innovation: A Study of Long Waves Economic Development* (London: Frances Pinter).

Friedman, M. and Friedman, R. (1980), *Free to Choose* (Harmondsworth: Penguin).

Friedson, E. (ed.) (1963), *The Hospital in Modern Society* (New York: Free Press/Macmillan).

Fuchs, V. R. (1986), *The Health Economy* (Cambridge, Mass.: Harvard University Press).

Fuchs, V. R. and Kramar, M. J. (1972), *Determinants of Expenditure for Physician Services in the United States 1948–1968*, National Bureau of Economic Research Occasional Paper, No. 117, DHEW Pub. no. (HSM) 73–3013 (Washington, DC: Department of Health, Education and Welfare).

Gehlen, A. (1980), *Man in the Age of Technology* (New York: Columbia University Press).

Gellner, E. (1987), *Culture, Identity, and Politics* (Cambridge: Cambridge University Press).

Gershuny, J. (1983a), *Social Innovation and the Division of Labour* (Oxford: Oxford University Press).

Gershuny, J. (1983b), 'Is Europe becoming a post-industrial society? Deindustrialization and the future of the service sector', in Braun *et al.* op. cit., pp. 118–37.

Gershuny, J. (1984), 'Growth, social innovation and time use', in Boulding, op. cit., pp. 36–59.

Gershuny, J. (1985), 'Towards a new social economics', in Roberts *et al.* op. cit., pp. 124–58.

Gershuny, J. and Miles, I. (1983), *The New Service Economy* (London: Frances Pinter).

Giddens, A. (1982), *Sociology: A Brief But Critical Introduction* (London: Macmillan).

Goodin, R. E. and Dryzak, J. (1987), 'Risk sharing and social justice: the motivational foundations of the post-war welfare state', in Goodin and LeGrand, op. cit., pp. 37–76.

Goodin, R. E., and LeGrand, J. (1987), *Not Only The Poor. The Middle Classes and the Welfare State* (London: Allen & Unwin).

Gosden, P. H. J. H. (1961), *The Friendly Societies in England 1815–1875* (Manchester: Manchester University Press).

Gough, I. (1979), *The Political Economy of the Welfare State* (London: Macmillan).

Grawbowski, H. G. (1980), 'Regulation and the international diffusion of pharmaceuticals', in Helms, op. cit., pp. 5–36.

Grabowski, H. G. and Vernon, J. M. (1982), 'The pharmaceutical industry', in Nelson, op. cit., pp. 282–360.

Gronbjerg, K. A. (1977), *Mass Society and the Extension of Welfare 1960–1970* (Chicago: University of Chicago Press).

Hall, J. A. (1981), *Diagnosis of Our Times: Six Views of Our Social Condition* (London: Heinemann).

Halmos, P. (1965), *The Faith of the Counsellors* (London: Hutchinson).

Hannah, L. (1986), *Inventing Retirement: The Development of Occupational Pensions in Britain* (Cambridge: Cambridge University Press).

Hawkins, S. W. (1988), *A Brief History of Time* (London: Bantam).

198   *References*

Heclo, H. (1974), *Modern Social Policies in Britain and Sweden: From Relief to Income Maintenance* (New Haven, Conn.: Yale University Press).

Heclo, H. (1981), 'Towards a new welfare state?', in Flora and Heidenheimer, op. cit., pp. 384–401.

Helms, R. R. (ed.) (1980), *The International Supply of Medicines. Implications of U.S. Regulatory Reform* (Washington, DC: American Enterprise Institute for Public Policy Research).

Henwood, F. and Thomas, G. (1984), *Science, Technology and Innovation. A Research Bibliography* (Brighton: Wheatsheaf).

Higgins, J. (1981), *States of Welfare. Comparative Analysis of Social Policy* (Oxford: Blackwell/Martin Robertson).

Higgins, J. (1988), *The Business of Medicine. Private Health Care in Britian* (London: Macmillan).

Hindess, B. (1987), *Equality, Freedom and the Market* (London: Tavistock).

Hollingsworth, J. R. (1986), *A Political Economy of Medicine: Great Britain and the United States* (Baltimore, Md: Johns Hopkins University Press).

Hollister, R. M., Kramer, B. M. and Bellin, S. S. (eds.) (1974), *Neighbourhood Health Centres* (Lexington, Mass.: Lexington).

Honigsbaum, F. (1979), *The Division in British Medicine: A History of the Separation of General Practice from Hospital Care 1911–1968* (London: Kogan Page).

Hough, G. W. (1975), *Technological Diffusion. Federal Programs and Procedures* (Mount Airy, Md.: Lomond).

Hummon, N. P. (1984), 'Organizational aspects of technological change', in Laudon, op. cit., pp. 67–81.

Isaac, L. and Kelly, W. R. (1981), 'Racial insurgency, the state, and the welfare expansion: local and national evidence from the postwar United States', *American Journal of Sociology*, vol. 86, no. 6, pp. 1348–86.

Jewkes, J., Sawers, D. and Stillerman, R. (1969), *The Sources of Invention*, 2nd edn (London: Macmillan).

Jones, K. (1972), *A History of the Mental Health Services* (London: Routledge & Kegan Paul).

Joyce, P. (1980), *Work, Society and Politics. The Culture of the Factory in Late Victorian England* (Brighton: Harvester).

Kenwood, A. G. and Lougheed, A. L. (1982), *Technological Diffusion and Industrialisation before 1914* (London/New York: Croom Helm/St Martins).

Kerr, C. (1983), *The Future of Industrial Societies. Convergence or Continuing Diversity?* (Cambridge, Mass.: Harvard University Press).

Kleinknicht, A. (1983), 'Observations on the Schumpeterian swarming of innovations', in Freeman, op. cit., pp. 48–61.

Kumar, K. (1978), *Prophecy and Progress. The Sociology of Industrial and Post-Industrial Society* (Harmondsworth: Penguin).

Larkin, G. (1983), *Occupational Monopoly and Modern Medicine* (London: Tavistock).

Laudon, R. (ed.) (1984), *The Nature of Technological Knowledge. Are Models of Scientific Change Relevant?* (Dordrecht: Reidel).

Law, S. A. (1974), *Blue Cross. What Went Wrong?* (New Haven, Conn.: Yale University Press).

Leavitt, J. W. (1986), *Brought to Bed: Childbearing in America, 1750–1950* (Oxford: Oxford University Press).

Leiby, J. (1978), *A History of Social Welfare and Social Work in the United States* (New York: Columbia University Press).

Levitt, R. (1977), *The Reorganised National Health Service*, 2nd edn (London: Croom Helm).

Liebenau, J. (1987), *Medical Science and Medical Industry. The Formation of the American Pharmaceutical Industry* (Baltimore, Md.: Johns Hopkins University Press).

Liem, R. (1981), 'Economic change and unemployment: contexts of illness', in Mishler *et al.*, op. cit., pp. 54–78.

Lundstedt, S. B. and Colglazier, E. W. (eds.) (1982), *Managing Innovation: The Social Dimensions of Creativity, Invention and Technology* (New York: Pergamon/Aspen Institute).

Mandel, E. (1980), *Long Waves of Capitalist Development* (Cambridge: Cambridge University Press).

Mandel, E. (1983), 'Explaining long waves of capitalist development', in Freeman, op. cit., pp. 195–202.

Mannor, T. R. and Morone, J. A. (1981), 'Innovation and the health services sector: notes on the United States', in Altenstetter, op. cit., pp. 35–42.

Mansfield, E. (1969), *The Economics of Technological Change* (London: Longman).

Mansfield, E., Rapoport, J., Romeo, A., Villani, E., Wagner, S. and Husie, F. (1977), *The Production and Application of New Industrial Technologies* (New York: Norton).

Markowitz, G. H. and Rosner, D. (1979), 'Doctors in crisis', in Reverby and Rosner, op. cit., pp. 185–205.

Marshall, T. H. (1965), *Social Policy* (London: Hutchinson).

Maxwell, R. J. (1981), *Health and Wealth. An International Study of Health Care Spending* (Lexington, Mass.: Lexington).

McKinley, J. B. (ed.) (1981), *Health Services Research, Planning and Change*, Milbank Reader vol. 4 (Cambridge, Mass.: MIT Press).

Mendelsohn, E., Swazey, J. P. and Taviss, I. (eds.) (1971), *Human Aspects of Innovation* (Cambridge, Mass.: Harvard University Press).

Mensch, G. (1979), *Stalemate in Technology. Innovations Overcome the Depression* (Cambridge, Mass.: Ballinger).

Mick, S. S. (1981), 'Understanding the persistence of human resource problems in health', in Mckinley, op. cit., pp. 83–119.

Miller, J. (1978), *The Body in Question* (London: Macmillan).

Miliband, R. (1969), *The State in Capitalist Society* (London: Weidenfeld & Nicolson).

Mishler, E. G. and AmaraSingham, L. R. (eds.) (1981), *Social Contexts of Health, Illness and Patient Care* (Cambridge: Cambridge University Press).

Mishra, R. (1977), *Society and Social Policy: Theoretical Perpectives on Welfare* (London: Macmillan).

Mishra, R. (1984), *The Welfare State in Crisis* (Brighton: Wheatsheaf).

Mobley, W. (1982), *Employee Turnover: Causes, Consequences and Control* (Reading, Mass.: Addison-Wesley).

Montgomery, D. (1979), *Workers' Control in America* (Cambridge: Cambridge University Press).

Morris, R. (1985), *Rethinking Social Welfare* (London/New York: Longman).

Mowday, R. T., Porter, L. W. and Steers, R. M. (1982), *Employee-Organization Linkages: The Psychology of Commitment, Absenteeism and Turnover* (New York: Academic).

Mulkay, M. J. (1972), *The Social Process of Innovation. A Study in the Sociology of Science* (London: Macmillan).

Nelson, R. R. (ed.) (1982), *Government and Technical Progress. A Cross Industry Perspective* (New York: Pergamon).

Nisbet, R. (1980), *History of the Idea of Progress* (London: Heinemann).

North, M. (1972), *The Secular Priests* (London: Allen & Unwin).

OECD, (1981), *The Welfare State in Crisis* (Paris: OECD).

OECD (1985a), *Measuring Health Care 1960–1983. Expenditure Costs and Performance*, Social Policy Studies No. 2 (Paris: OECD).

OECD (1985b), *Social Expenditure 1960–1990. Problems of Growth and Control* (Paris: OECD).

Offe, C. (1984), *Contradictions of the Welfare State* (London: Hutchinson).

Osherson, S. and AmaraSingham, L. (1981), 'The machine metaphor in medicine', in Mishler *et al.*, op. cit., pp. 218–49.

Pacey, A. (1983), *The Culture of Technology* (Oxford: Blackwell).

Perrow, C. (1979), 'Goals and power structures. A historical case study', in Reverby and Rosner, op. cit., pp. 112–46.

Pickstone, J. (1985), *Medicine and Industrial Society: A History of Hospital Development in Manchester and its Region, 1752–1946* (Manchester: Manchester University Press).

Pinker, R. (1971), *Social Theory and Social Policy* (London: Heinemann).

Polsky, N. W. (1984), *Policy Innovation in America: The Politics of Initiation* (New Haven, Conn.: Yale University Press).

Proceedings of the 1977 Sun Valley Forum on National Health Care (1979), *Medical Technology: The Culprit Behind Health Care Cost*

Increases, DHEW Pub. No. (PHS) 79–3216 (Washington, DC: US Department of Health, Education and Welfare).

Rau, N. (1974), *Trade Cycles: Theory and Evidence*, Studies in Economics (London: Macmillan).

Ray, G. F. (1984), *The Diffusion of Mature Technologies*, National Institute for Social and Economic Research Occasional Paper, No. XXXVI, (Cambridge: Cambridge University Press).

Reekie, W. D. (1975), *The Economics of the Pharmaceutical Industry* (London: Macmillan).

Rein, M. (1983), *From Policy to Practice* (London: Macmillan).

Reiser, S. J. (1978), *Medicine and the Reign of Technology* (New York: Cambridge University Press).

Reverby, S. (1979), 'The search for the hospital yardstick: nursing and the rationalization of hospital work', in Reverby and Rosner, op. cit., pp. 206–25.

Reverby, S. and Rosner, D. (eds.) (1979), *Health Care in America* (Philadelphia, Pa.: Temple University Press).

Richardson, J. T. (1945), *The Origin and Development of Group Hospitalization in the United States* (Columbia, Miss.: University of Missouri Press).

Rimlinger, G. (1971), *Welfare Policy and Industrialisation in Europe, America and Russia* (New York: Wiley).

Ritter, G. A. (1986), *Social Welfare in Germany and Britain* (Leamington Spa/New York: Berg).

Roberts, B., Finnegan, R. and Gallie, D. (eds.) (1985), *New Approaches to Economic Life: Economic Restructuring, Unemployment and the Social Division of Labour* (Manchester: Manchester University Press).

Roberts, D. (1960), *Victorian Origins of the British Welfare State* (New Haven, Conn.: Yale University Press).

Roberts, D. (1979), *Paternalism in Early Victorian England* (London: Croom Helm).

Rogers, E. M. (1983), *Diffusion of Innovations*, 3rd edn (New York: Free Press).

Rose, M. (1972), *The Relief of Poverty 1834–1914*, Studies in Economic History (London: Macmillan).

Rosen, G. (1963), 'The hospital. Historical sociology of a community institution', in Friedson, op. cit., pp. 1–36.

Rosner, D. (1979), 'Business of the bedsick: health care in Brooklyn', in Reverby and Rosner, op. cit., pp. 117–31.

Rostow, W. W. (1983), 'Scarcity and abundance of foodstuffs and raw materials', in Freeman, op. cit., pp. 13–25.

Rothwell, R. and Zegveld, W. (1981), *Industrial Innovation and Public Policy* (London: Frances Pinter).

Routh, G. (1980), *Occupation and Pay in Great Britain 1906–1979*, 2nd edn (London: Macmillan).

Rule, J. B. (1978), *Insight and Social Betterment. A Preface to Applied Social Science* (New York: Oxford University Press).

Russell, L. B. (1979), *Technology in Hospitals: Medical Advances and their Diffusion* (Washington, DC.: Brookings Institution).

Rutstein, D. D. (1967), *The Coming Revolution in Medicine* (Cambridge, Mass.: MIT Press).

Ruttan, V. W. (1959), 'Usher and Schumpeter on invention, innovation and technological change', *Quarterly Journal of Economics*, vol. 73, pp. 596–606.

Scherer, F. M. (1984), *Innovation and Growth. Schumpeterian Perspectives* (Cambridge, Mass.: MIT Press).

Schroeder, S. S. and Showstack, J. A. (1979), 'Medical technology: the culprit behind rising health costs', in Proceedings of the 1977 Sun Valley Forum on National Health Costs, op. cit., pp. 178–212.

Shryock, R. H. (1960), *Medicine and Society in America 1660–1860* (New York: New York University Press).

Sidel, V. (1971), 'New technologies and the practice of medicine', in Mendelsohn, Swazey and Taviss, op. cit., pp. 131–55.

Singelmann, J. and Tienda, M. (1985), 'The process of occupational change in a service society: the case of the U.S.', in Roberts *et al.*, op. cit., pp. 48–67.

Smith, F. B. (1979), *The People's Health 1830–1910* (London: Croom Helm).

Starr, P. (1982), *The Social Transformation of American Medicine: The Rise of a Sovereign Profession and the Making of a Vast Industry* (New York: Basic Books).

Stevens, R. and Stevens, R. (1974), *Welfare Medicine in America. A Case Study of Medicaid* (New York: Free Press).

Stoman, D. F. (1976), *The Medical Establishment and Social Responsibility* (New York: Kennikat Press).

Stoneman, P. (1983), *The Economic Analysis of Technological Change* (New York: Oxford University Press).

Stonier, T. (1983), *The Wealth of Information* (London: Methuen).

Stroeckle, J. D. and Candib, L. M. (1974), 'The neighbourhood health center. Reform ideas of yesterday and today', in Hollister, Kramer and Bellin, op. cit., pp. 25–40.

de Swaan, A. (1988), *In the Care of the State* (New York: Oxford University Press).

Tarr, J. A., McCurley J., McMichael, F. C. and Yosie, T., (1984), 'Water and wastes: a retrospective assessment of wastewater technology in the United States, 1800–1932', *Technology and Culture*, vol. 25, no. 2, pp. 226–63.

Taylor-Gooby, P. (1983), 'The distributional compulsion and the moral order of the welfare state', in Ellis and Kumar, op. cit., pp. 98–121.

Teeling-Smith, G. (ed.) (1980a), *The Pharmaceutical Industry and Society* (London: Office of Health Economics).

Teeling-Smith, G. (1980b), 'Social and economic pressures in the pharmaceutical industry', in Teeling-Smith, op. cit., pp. 89–107.

Titmuss, R. M. (1974), *Social Policy* (London: Allen & Unwin).

Titmuss, R. M. (1976), *Essays on the Welfare State*, 3rd edn (London: Allen & Unwin).

Toffler, A. (1980), *The Third Wave* (London: Collins).

Towler, J. and Bramall, J. (1986), *Midwives in History and Society* (London: Croom Helm).

Townsend, P. (1976), *Sociology and Social Policy* (Harmondsworth: Penguin).

Trease, G. E. (1964), *Pharmacy in History* (London: Ballière, Tindall & Cox).

Usher, A. P. (1954), *A History of Mechanical Invention*, rev. edn (New Haven, Conn.: Harvard University Press).

Uttley, S. (1980), 'The welfare exchange reconsidered', *Journal of Social Policy*, vol. 9, no. 2, pp. 187–205.

Uttley, S. (1984), 'Reformulating the development theory of welfare', *Journal of Social Policy*, vol. 13, no. 4, pp. 447–65.

Vaughan, P. (1970), *The Pill on Trial* (Harmondsworth: Penguin).

Verbrugge, V. H. (1979), 'The social meaning of personal health', in Reverby and Rosner, op. cit., pp. 45–66.

Vogel, M. J. (1979), 'The transformation of the American hospital', in Reverby and Rosner, op. cit., pp. 105–16.

Vogel, M. J. (1980), *The Invention of the Modern Hospital* (Chicago: University of Chicago Press).

Waddington, I. (1973), 'The role of the hospital in the development of modern medicine', *Sociology*, vol. 7, pp. 211–23.

Wallace, A. F. C. (1982), *The Social Context of Innovation. Bureaucrats, Families and Heroes in the Early Industrial Revolution as Foreseen in Bacon's New Atlantis* (Princeton, NJ: Princeton University Press).

Watkin, B. (1978), *The National Health Service: The First Phase 1848–1974* (London: Allen & Unwin).

Watson, J. B. (1981), *The Double Helix: A Personal Account of the Discovery of the Structure of DNA* (London: Weidenfeld & Nicolson).

Wildavsky, A. (1982), 'Progress and public policy', in Almond *et al.*, op. cit., pp. 361–74.

Wilensky, H. (1975), *The Welfare State and Equality* (Berkeley, Calif.: University of California Press).

Williams, T. I. (1982), *A Short History of 20th Century Technology* (Oxford: Oxford University Press).

Wohl, A. S. (1983), *Endangered Lives. Public Health in Victorian Britain* (London: Dent).

Woodward, J. (1974), *To Do the Sick No Harm. A Study of the British Voluntary Hospital System to 1875* (London: Routledge & Kegan Paul).

Woodward, J. (1984), 'Medicine and the city: the nineteenth-century experience', in Woods and Woodward, op. cit., pp. 65–78.

Woods, R. and Woodward, J. (eds.) (1984), *Urban Disease and Mortality in Nineteenth Century England* (London/New York: Batsford/St Martins Press).

Wootton, B. (1983), 'Reflections on the welfare state', in Bean and MacPherson, op. cit., pp. 282–93.

Youngson, A. J. (1979), *The Scientific Revolution in Victorian Medicine* (London: Croom Helm).

Additional Reading

Abel-Smith, B., *A History of the Nursing Profession* (London: Heinemann, 1960).

Anderson, O. W., *The Uneasy Equilibrium. Private and Public Financing of Health Services in the United States 1875–1965* (New Haven, Conn.: College and University Press, 1968).

Archer, M. S., *Social Origins of Education Systems* (London: Sage, 1979).

Aron, R., *The Industrial Society* (London: Weidenfeld & Nicolson, 1967).

Aron, R., *Progress and Disillusion: The Dialectics of Modern Society* (Harmondsworth: Penguin, 1968).

Ashford, D. E. (ed.), *Comparing Public Policies: New Concepts and Methods* (Beverly Hills, Calif.: Sage, 1978).

Axin, J. and Levin, H., *Social Welfare: A History of the American Response to Need* (New York: Harper & Row, 1975).

Baly, M. E., *Florence Nightingale and the Nursing Legacy* (London: Croom Helm, 1986).

Berliner, H., *A System of Scientific Medicine* (London: Tavistock, 1985).

Brockington, C. F., *A Short History of Public Health* (London: Churchill, 1966).

Checkland, S., *British Public Policy 1776–1939: An Economic, Social and Political Perspective* (Cambridge: Cambridge University Press, 1983).

Checkoway, B., *Citizens and Health Care* (New York: Pergamon, 1981).

Clarke, F. H. (ed.), *How Modern Medicines are Discovered* (New York: Futura, 1973).

Coleman, J. S., *Medical Innovation: A Diffusion Study* (Indianapolis, Ind.: Bobbs Merrill, 1966).

Coll, B. D., *Perspectives in Public Welfare: A History* (Washington, DC: US Department of Health, Education and Welfare, 1969).

Cooper, M. H., *Prices and Profits in the Pharmaceutical Industry* (Oxford: Pergamon, 1966).

Crowther, M. A., *British Social Policy, 1914–1939* (London: Macmillan, 1987).

Davis, K. and Schren, C., *Health and the War on Poverty. A Ten Year Appraisal* (Washington, DC.: Brookings Institution, 1978).

Evers, A., Nowotny, H. and Wintersberger, H., *The Changing Face of Welfare* (Aldershot: Gower, 1987).

Flora, P., 'Solution or source of crisis? The welfare state in historical perspective', in Mommsen, op. cit., pp. 343–89.
Fraser, D., *The Evolution of the British Welfare State*, 2nd edn (London: Macmillan, 1984).
Fulkson, J., *HMOs and the Politics of Health System Reform* (Chicago: American Hospitals Association, 1980).

Gellner, E., *Thought and Change* (London: Weidenfeld & Nicolson, 1964).
Gilbert, N., *Capitalism and the Welfare State: Dilemmas of Social Benevolence* (New Haven, Conn.: Yale University Press, 1985).
Greer, A. L., 'Advances in the study of diffusion of innovation in health', *Milbank Memorial Quarterly*, vol. 55, 1977, pp. 505–632.
Grossman, M., *The Demand for Health. A Theoretical and Empirical Investigation* (New York: National Bureau for Economic Research, 1972).

Hall, P., 'The geography of the fifth Kondratieff cycle', *New Society* 26 March 1981, pp. 535–7.
Handler, J. F., *Reforming the Poor: Welfare Policy, Federalism and Morality* (New York: Basic, 1972).
Harvard University Program on Technology and Society, *Technology and Social History*, Research Review No. 8 (Cambridge, Mass.: Harvard University Press, 1971).
Hasenfield, Y., and Zald, M. N., *The Welfare State in America. Trends and Prospects* (Beverly Hills, Calif.: Sage, 1985).
Heidenheimer, A. J., Heclo, H. and Teisch, A. C., *Comparative Public Policy: The Politics of Social Change in Europe and America* (London: Macmillan, 1975).

Inglis, B., *Drugs, Doctors and Disease* (London: André Deutsch, 1965).

Jones, C., *Patterns of Social Policy: An Introduction to Comparative Analysis* (London: Tavistock, 1985).

Katz, E., 'The social itinerary of technical change: two studies in diffusion of innovation', *Human Organization*, vol. 10, no. 2, 1961, pp. 210–33.
Kerr, C., *et al.*, *Industrialism and Industrial Man* (Harmondsworth: Penguin, 1973).

King, L. S., *Medical Thinking: A Historical Preface* (Princeton, NJ: Princeton University Press, 1982).

Klein, R. and O'Higgins, M., *The Future of Welfare* (Oxford: Blackwell, 1985).

Langendonck, J. van, *Prelude to Harmony on a Community Theme: Health Care Insurance in the Six and Britain* (Oxford: Oxford University Press, 1975).

Leichter, H. M., *A Comparative Approach to Policy Analysis: Health Care Policy in Four Nations* (Cambridge: Cambridge University Press, 1979).

Luft, H. S., *Health Maintenance Organizations: Dimensions of Performance* (New York: Wiley, 1981).

Maitra, P., *Population, Technology and Development* (Aldershot: Gower, 1986).

Marshall, R. A. and Zubay, E. A., *The Debit System of Marketing Life and Health Insurance* (Engelwood Cliffs, NJ: Prentice-Hall, 1975).

Mathews, R. C., Feinstein, C. H. and Odling-Smee, J., *et al.*, *British Economic Growth 1856–1973* (Stanford: Stanford University Press, 1982).

McKeown, T., *Medicine in Modern Society* (London: Allen & Unwin, 1965).

McKinley, J. B. (ed.), *Politics and Health Care*, Milbank Reader No. 6, (Cambridge, Mass.: MIT Press, 1981).

McLachlan, G. and McKeown, T. (eds.), *Medical History and Medical Care* (Oxford: Oxford University Press, 1971).

Mommsen, W. J., *The Emergence of the Welfare State in Britain and Germany* (London: Croom Helm, 1981).

Moon, M. (ed.), *Economic Transfers in the United States*, Studies in Income and Wealth No. 49, (Chicago: National Bureau of Economic Research/University of Chicago Press, 1975).

Morantz-Sanchez, R. M., *Sympathy and Science: Women Physicians in American Medicine* (New York: Oxford University Press, 1986).

Navarro, V., *Class Struggle, the State and Medicine* (London: Martin Robertson, 1978).

OECD, *Public Expenditure on Health* (Paris: OECD, 1977).

Parker, J. E. S., *The Economics of Innovation, The National and Multinational Enterprise in Technological Change* (London: Longman, 1978).

Rifkin, J., *Entropy. A New World View* (New York: Viking, 1980).

Rosenberg, N., *Inside the Black Box: Technology and Economics* (Cambridge: Cambridge University Press, 1982).

Rostow, W. R., *The Barbaric Counter Revolution* (Austin, Tex.: University of Texas Press, 1983).

Social Security Administration, Office of Research and Statistics, *The Size and Shape of the Medical Dollar*, DHEW Pub. No. (SSA) 73–119, (Washington, DC.: U.S. Department of Health, Education and Welfare, 1972).

Taylor, R., *Medicine Out of Control. The Anatomy of a Malignant Technology* (Melbourne: Sun Books, 1979).

Taverner, D., *The Impending Medical Revolution* (London: Hodder & Stoughton, 1968).

Trattner, W. I., *From Poor Law to Welfare State* (New York: Macmillan, 1974).

Waldman, S., *The Effect of Changing Technology on Hospital Costs* Research and Statistics Note No. 4, (Washington, DC.: US Department of Health, Education and Welfare, Social Security Administration, 1972).

Weindling, P., *The Social History of Occupational Health* (London: Croom Helm, 1985).

Wildavsky, A., 'Doing better and feeling worse', *Daedalus*, Winter 1977, pp. 105–23.

Woodward, J. and Richards, D., *Health Care and Popular Medicine in 19th Century England* (London: Croom Helm, 1977).

Index

THE LIBRARY
UNIVERSITY OF CALIFORNIA
San Francisco
(415) 476-2335

THIS BOOK IS DUE ON THE LAST DATE STAMPED BELOW

Books not returned on time are subject to fines according to the Library Lending Code. A renewal may be made on certain materials. For details consult Lending Code.

6 WEEK LOAN